Exercise
Motivational Triggers

Exercise Motivational Triggers

Be Your Own Personal Trainer

Dave Baldwin

Writer's Showcase
San Jose New York Lincoln Shanghai

Exercise Motivational Triggers
Be Your Own Personal Trainer

Writer's Showcase
an imprint of iUniverse, Inc.

For information address:
iUniverse, Inc.
5220 S. 16th St., Suite 200
Lincoln, NE 68512
www.iuniverse.com

Consult your doctor prior to beginning any new exercise program.

ISBN: 0-595-21603-X

Printed in the United States of America

*I want to thank those we have lost, those we have found, those who dream
and those who lend hope the dreamers.
I dedicate this to the loving memory of my father and those other special
family members who have passed.
I thank
Mom, Joey, Gigi, Susan, Paul and Ralph for their insights.
Finally, I thank
my wonderful son David and Andrea.*

Contents

Preface

Does This Dream Sound Familiar?

"Here I am. I've finally done it! My body feels better than it did when I was eighteen. This really is my kind of day. Nothing will keep me from doing what I want or from being whom I want. I am motivated and ready for action. Oh look, another mirror. I really look too good to pass-by a mirror without seeing all that I have become. Across the room, I can see those young bathing beauties staring-me-down, again. I guess I will give them a thrill and pass their way. Some days I just cannot decide what, of all the wonderful things I am, is the best part. When I stop to think, that I use to lie on the sofa every weekend, wishing I looked better and felt better. I am so happy I discovered my motivation and got moving. Oh wait; there is that blonde coming-over to me. I will bet she wants…(LICK)…what the…?"

Suddenly you are awakened by your loving pet licking you on the face, as your loving bride has trained him to do when you have been napping on the sofa too long. Don't you hate it when that happens? In your dreams you are on the verge of God-like potential. You feel as though you belong on Mount Olympus. While, in reality, you have been spending almost every weekend, of the past 850, procrastinating. You have outdone yourself with procrastination. You have become an expert. It would be an easy bet that you even impressed yourself with your ability to procrastinate.

Perhaps this sounds more familiar. "No, no, I better just wait here in my chair (All men have "their" chair. We don't know why.) Someone may call. There may be someone else who is doing nothing tonight, just like me. 'Yup', I better just settle-in to my easy chair. No! Wait! The sofa, yea, the sofa would be much better. That will get the job done. Besides, who am I to try and change my world overnight? And wait one more minute. I remember there is a great movie on tonight. If I wanted to exercise, I would have to get-up, go all the way to the bedroom, change cloths, and lord forbid, have to go outside in that unbearable 80-degree heat. (For those of us in towns like Houston, TX, 80 degrees in the summer would be a dream come true.) It would even be worse if I wanted to drive to the fitness center. Those 3 miles are killers. This sofa is best for me. I need my rest. Those 6 hour work days 3 days a week will really drain a guy."

As George Carlin would suggest, find the humor in everything. Everyone is encouraged to find the humor in the whole exercise industry. I feel humor keeps life in perspective. Further, I think humor is one of the tools I have always employed when teaching people about exercise. Humor tempers our fitness goals and allows fun to be part of any new exercise endeavor. Exercise, health and beauty is a multi-billion dollar industry because we all want "it" (health and beauty). The people who get "it" pay with sweat and financial equity. Those who seek health and beauty with only financial means are fooling themselves. This book is far more about living healthfully than seeking the perfect body. Again, poking fun at the whole ideal of perfect bodies allows appropriate perspective on our true individual physical potentials. When you discover how to take a joke, you will spend far more time laughing with people, than being the brunt of the joke.

This book is about hope, potential, a tool, dispelling myths and having fun with it all. There is no "magic pill", without consequence, no optimal plan that fits all. One size does not fit all. The only magic happens when someone takes action to be better than they were yesterday.

We all carry the potential for magic—exercising blessings. Whether we are bettering ourselves or someone else, it is always a blessing to be thankful for. Even in failure, there is blessing.

Remember your past "fitness failures" for the education they are worth. I can recall a friend's idea of fitness failures. She told me of the times she would spend months in a regular exercise program. She would eat right and exercise often. She would lose fat and inches. She would begin to enjoy the way she felt and how she looked. Then, after breaking-up with a boyfriend, changing jobs or simply getting caught in a cycle of eating too much, she would find herself, months later, bigger and wider than she was before. Obviously, her goal of maintaining her healthier body was not achieved. Failure without learning is just painful; however, failure that spawns education and improvement brings you closer to success. It has been said by many, in many ways, that the person who never fails is doing nothing. The Dalai Lama says, "Often people ask me what is the quickest method [to gain enlightenment], the fastest, and, in their minds I think, what is the cheapest. This is the sign of failure. If the goal is worth achieving, don't think about those things." Whether seeking enlightenment or something less cerebral such as a better body, appropriate effort is required. With that ideal, it could be suggested, that as long as we learn from our mistakes, failure does not exist. Any plan to achieve better health requires a great deal of effort, sacrifice and, more importantly, effort.

After reading this, some would certainly tell me I must be "full of it". I know people who would argue both sides of that argument. That aside, I encourage you to view those times you have stumbled, as trials you endured. If you believe that personal trials equal learning, then the more trials you have, the more you learn. Thus, we must endure the education of failure to produce greater and greater potential for success.

Consider Thomas Edison, who tried more than eight thousand filaments before he found one that would last. That is right. Look at the nearest light bulb and thank old Tom under breath. Crazy or not, Mr. Edison never gave-up. While you are speaking under your breath, take a moment to thank yourself for trying again to be better. By opening this volume, you are trying to find the "motivation trigger" which might help you get the physique and heart you want. The vast majority of what you need to achieve the lofty physical goals you want is staring back at you in every mirror you see. Corny as that last statement may sound, sometimes, corny works.

Why Exercise?

Having a stronger body can help improve a poor mental state. Please do not take my word for it. If you want to read what the researchers and educators have found, you will find them listed in the references section.

**************** Blah, Blah, Blah...I can give you physiological reasons why a stronger body helps the mental processes. So what if exercise has been found to increase dopamine, serotonin and nor epinephrine (commonly referred to as the "antidepressant hormones") in the body. The truth is most people do not care about all the supporting research, as long as they get the **results** they desire—the bottom-line. Without getting bogged-down in the science of exercise, it is still important to consider the existing tie between the body, mind and spirit (the big three).

If one takes-stock in the spirit, mind and body concept, then one would believe that those three elements are never really separate. These elements are continuously intermingling, relying on the others to be complements. As if working-out with a training partner, some days the mind carries the body and the spirit, while on other days it is the spirit or body carrying the other two. We all have our weaknesses and our strengths. Sometimes the lines separating the three elements blur—we begin by exercising one element, meanwhile feeding the others—the body, mind or spirit. We never help one of the big three without helping the complement.

During one of the toughest points in my life, I challenged my body to carry a mind beaten-down by the demands of an unmanageable irreparable situation. When I faced a pending divorce to a woman I continued to love, I did not know how to manage my pain. My divorce was easily the hardest thing I have ever endured. Compared to some, what I endured was far less. Whether you are the grand champion of pain endurance, or have had the easiest life ever, everyone needs help sometimes. My help and solace was found in physical activity, general activity, exercising the mind and feeding a weak spirit. Always remember, that the spirit, mind and the body never operate with complete independence of one another.

When I found my moments of despair consuming, it was exercise that brought me back—back to my basic gifts. Each of us has gifts, which are meant to be shared with those we touch. My passion for exercise is my gift. Exercise became a tool, used throughout my tougher times, working to try and keep my mind focused forward. There are poor choices—temptations that take us off the path that can sedate dedication to a healthy lifestyle. With my divorce, everyday my heart would break a little more, hopes would fade, depression would loom, and the baron horizon came closer. I did not know how to let go of love, move forward and find the new horizon? I learned quickly that, just as you cannot see the finish line with your head down, you cannot see the horizon until you climb above the peak. My road to healing started when I began to care for my body while the mind and the spirit tried to heal. Yes, the spirit must heal also. God can and will heal it, if you ask. Please be reminded, that we not only ask for healing through prayer, we also ask for healing by living by God's word.

Like many, I went through times when I questioned my faith, feeling as prayers had gone unanswered. When we question our faith, we must challenge the body to change, feeling the exhilaration of physical strength. From physical power, mental strength is fostered and the spirit can sore. Since all we have is gifted from God, the physical work we do is another way to exercise the spirit. It is time to believe the unfolding of reality and accept God's will. Sometimes what we pray for is not what is best for all. God knows what is best. Sometimes God gives us what we need, which may not be what we pray for. I found the worst pain I had ever known. Not even the loss of my father affected me like this loss of love. From this pain, I was able to release control and take a leap of faith. I also realize life can be long, and to think my suffering on earth has hit its peak would be naive. I cannot explain away, justify or minimize this. For me shadows loomed, blanketing a family—my family. Families thrive on a thin line of vows, commitment, love, and devotion. When lost, these elements fade together as an **amalgimous** mass, immaterial as any promise not kept. Wow, that sounds like pretty heavy stuff. Now what? My family was a wreck, and I felt like crap. Now what?

What is the bottom-line, you might ask? For me, the challenges inherent in divorce served as great motivation to exercise. For others, it would be a reason to do many other things. The only promises we control are those we make to others or, more importantly, to ourselves.

I close this section with a few words from Dr. Wayne Dyer. Although not stronger than the bible, his writings and insights are some of the things that helped me persevere through trying times. "Enlightenment is the quiet acceptance of what is. If we are to have magical bodies, we must have magical minds. Judgment means that you view the world as you are, rather than it is." (Dr. Wayne W. Dyer, Dr. Wayne W. *Everyday Wisdom.* Carson, CA: Hay House, Inc., 1993). Dr. Wayne Dyer is one of the most widely read internationally best-selling authors in the field of personal development. When Dr. Dyer speaks about accepting things, I believe you give-over to it. Give-over to what "is". As the bible tells us, lay your burdens at the foot of the cross. Through him, all things are possible. Let his majesty raise your chin to face the day anew.

This book is a symbol of my journey back to health and happiness on the tails of what I know best in life—exercise. I thought I knew more about women than I do. So, exercise it is…

You will be taken through all the steps I use when helping anyone develop an exercise program. My goal is to always show people how to get the results they want. It should not be about how physically fit we are, but how happy and healthy we are. If we can raise your self-esteem, prevent illness, improve stamina, etc., then great. However, if you are still not enjoying life more, as a result of improving your physical self, there is something missing. Exercise is obviously not a cure for all moods and difficult times in our lives. In any disparaging time, additional professional help from the fields of psychology, medicine and clergy, should always be considered. One of your other elements, the spirit or mind, may need some specific care for lasting improvement. Having a sense of peace and a feeling of WELLNESS are vital in life.

Introduction

Before you begin to exercise, it is important to create the proper amount of perspective on this new effort. Let us begin by exercising your funny bone. A friend sent me the 10 best reasons for not exercising. The author was anonymous. Forget the drudgery that regular exercise can be and remember it can be fun also.

As you read, see if you can identify with any of these.

10—My grandmother started walking five miles a day when she was 60. She's 97 now and we don't know where in the hell she is.

9—The only reason I would start jogging is so that I could hear heavy breathing again.

8—I joined a health club last year, spent 400 bucks and haven't lost a pound. Apparently you have to show-up.

7—I have to exercise in the morning before my brain figures-out what I'm doing.

6—I don't exercise at all. If God meant us to touch our toes, he would have put them further up our body.

5—I like long walks, especially when they are taken by people who annoy me.

4—I have flabby thighs, but fortunately my stomach covers them.

3—The advantage of exercising every day is that you die healthier.

2—If you are going to try cross-country skiing, start with a small country.

1—I don't jog. It makes the ice jump right out of my glass.

Conversely, hear are 10 great reasons to exercise.

Exercise helps;
Increase your self-confidence and self-esteem
Improve your digestion
You to sleep better
Give you more energy
Enable you to lose weight and keep it off
Build strength
Improve endurance
Enhance, coordination and balance
Strengthen your bones
Enrich sexuality

The general reasons for regular exercise are far more numerous than what we have just listed. Find your reason and get into it.

For Success in Exercise—Find your reason!!!!!!!!!
Ann could have easily been described as an advertiser's dream. Every new piece of exercise equipment on the market was the perceived key to her successful transformation from "fat" to "fit". She bought treadmills, ski machines, abdominal exercisers, elastic bands, ankle weights, etc. Ann loved the wonderful world of fitness magic. "Just five minutes a day can turn you into the Goddess you always wanted to be." Come on! Ok, I know this sounds condescending, but isn't it true? People want the magic pill to save them from themselves—overeating and being lazy. Living 1400 miles from Ann, I did not know what the latest scheme was for her weight management. She came to visit me about eight months after starting her latest program. I picked up Ann at the airport, and almost did not recognize her. She had lost 30 pounds and had her asthma under control. You see, I had spent years sharing effective weight management strategies

with Ann. I wanted for her, more than anyone else in her life, to feel stronger and healthier. Yet, Ann kept turning to the latest and greatest, opposed to the tried and true. It was not until she employed proven techniques of dietary control and exercise persistence, that she achieved the results she so deeply desired. You see, Ann is Ann Baldwin, my mother. I believe she had a difficult time seeing her youngest child as the accomplished exercise professional he had become. I can see her saying to herself, "Wait, you were just my little boy, how could you consult me on a professional exercise program?" I could respond with, "Well, you see Mom, you sent me to school, gave me books and led me to a path of knowledge." When you study and practice something for more than 20 years, you retain a few things. I am thankful that most people listened more intently than my mother, people such as Jim.

Jim was well overweight and needing to lose more than 50 pounds. To put it simply, he followed a safe and effective plan he and I developed. Jim had never been involved in a regular exercise program. He had realized his own professional and financial success, and now wanted to achieve physical success. I set him to task, and Jim set to work shortly after our first meeting. Not long after that meeting I took a new job across town. Some months later I went back to the old job, and saw Jim. Jim had lost more than 40 pounds following the simplest of plans—a plan of effort and progression. You would not have believed the positive change in Jim. He exuded confidence and enthusiasm I had not seen when he began the program we developed. Obviously, everyone will not achieve the results Jim did, nor should they. His goals were personal, just as yours should be. Jim proved the determination he spoke of in that initial meeting. Not only was he determined, he faced his fear of failure with a wide-eyed and realistic view of himself.

If you have not already begun to consider your real motivation to begin a regular exercise program, please do it now. The appropriate motivation should be clear before digesting and utilizing what you extract from this text. No matter the exercise program you choose, it will fail if you begin with half-hearted intentions. Whatever your "motivational triggers", remember and befriend them for the guiding light they provide. I wish you luck in your quests for health and peace.

Chapter 1

Pulling Apart The Person

There is no greater barrier to physical activity than you. Baring severe, paralyzing health situations, there is no greater barrier to getting active than ourselves. The mind tells you what it wants. The body tells the mind what it needs. We are physical creatures, born to hunt. Since grocery stores and restaurants supply the harvest, and the kill, hunting ain't what it used to be.

Be as honest with yourself as possible. Stop finding justification for your shortcomings or the poor choices you have made. The mental exercise in this chapter is less about reflection, and more about what you do with the next second of your future.

Someone dear to me spent many years criticizing my tendency to be introspective. I am telling you right now, that introspection is about searching the past to be better in the future. If someone criticizes you for it, it can only be for two reasons, either they lack the ability to do it, or they don't like what they see when they are introspective. What do you see when you look inside? To be introspective you have to challenge your own perception. Can you really put yourself in the other person's shoes? Can you understand why your spouse yelled at you? Can you see that sometimes it is not a personal attack, but a lashing-out based on circumstance? If you can't see these things, you have not found introspection. If you are most concerned about how that person makes you feel, as opposed to how they feel, or what your role was in getting to that moment, you are not challenging your own perception.

A member of a fitness center once told me that they would not go into the fitness center they had joined when certain persons were there. They justify this action by saying, "They make me uncomfortable. They try to help me in ways I don't want to be helped." For goodness sake, if you have a problem, speak up. **Be assertive enough to exercise the control you have to create the environment you need to get the results you want.** Do not use how another person acts as an excuse. If you want help or you don't like what someone says, ask them to help or refrain. If you treat it as a confrontation, it is. If you treat it as an unassuming suggestion, it can be taken that way. Your comfort with one or two people, outside of harassment, of hundreds of members, should never keep you from the exercise schedule you want. If this is happening, it is your fault—your perception.

Our lifestyles are choices we make. You and I make choices everyday, to get fit, to be productive, to avoid discussions or **not**! Our perceptions, which can result in barriers, are the real obstacles in life. Research by the American College of Sports Medicine reports that the greatest obstacle to regular exercise people reported was a lack of time. **Here it is,…we find the time for what we value most.** To be realistic for a moment, we must all take care of the essentials in life, such as food, shelter and family. This discussion is not an attempt to belittle the priorities people set before exercise. Rather, this discussion is about accepting what we want most. On behalf of everyone you complain to, whining about not having enough time to exercise is a cop-out. Do you know how many people play the same tired song in their head every day? As long as you continue telling yourself, you have no time, you do not and will not. On the other hand, if you plan your schedule to commit time to an exercise regime, you improve your chances for success. When do we become the higher priority in our schedules? Time is truly a precious commodity, to be managed carefully.

This is not intended to give you all kinds of strategies for time management. The focus here is on personal priorities, perceived value of exercise and being honest with yourself. Do not waste all your time reciting the laundry list of reasons why your schedule is so busy. Sometimes you have to just start moving—do something. Write the first line. Throw the first pitch. Hit the first ball. If you walked for a minute today, do two the next day, and so on. When do you want to start feeling better, looking better and just being better?

Many people work in industries that require constant contact with their company, as a vendor in the medical industry would be. These vendors wear a pager 24 hours a day, 7 days a week. Quickly, I want to breakdown their barriers to regular exercise for you. First, there are similar patterns that emerge, even in this line of work. They usually have to be at work before 9:00am only 2 to 3 days a week. This gives them 2 to 3 mornings a week to walk or do calisthenics. For those with kids, the kids could ride bikes while they walk, before taking them to school. If they need to make some of the many phone calls needed in the day, they can take the phone on the walk. In their typical day, mornings are the most predictable times to use for exercise.

Do you see the insignificant obstacles we choose to place in front of ourselves? Try not to mistake opportunities for obstacles.

Let's take another case scenario. Jane and Bob work two jobs each, volunteer several times each month for a local organization, share two beautiful children from Bob's previous marriage 6 days per month. Both people work hard and play hard. Yet, both want to feel better, be more fit and lose some weight. Bob has access to several exercise centers through his job. Jane has similar access to exercise centers through Bob. They see each other at least two evenings a week and both weekend days. There are at least 4 days a week they could be walking together. There are seven mornings they could do 20 or 30 minutes of easy calisthenics exercise. They have a half dozen different exercise videos, showing many different exercises.

And yet, with all the tools, time and circumstance, they still do not exercise.

We can be our greatest source of motivation or our greatest source of barriers. As long as you look outside yourself—there is always a reason to be lazy. If you pull apart yourself, open-up, face the day with an open mind and heart, what will you find? Many of us may not like what we see at times, for the choices we have made, or people we think we have become.

It is time to discover your true barriers to a regular active lifestyle.

These are the TOP 10 reasons I have heard from people, as to why they do not exercise on a regular basis:

No time—Too Busy
No money
No place
No Child Care
Injury
No doctor's approval
Don't know what to do
No partner
Too out of shape
Hate exercise
Too Hard—This would be on the list, but most egos don't like to admit it.

Do any of these fit you? Perhaps, you have compiled your own comprehensive list? Whatever your reasons for not exercising may be, I have developed my own rebuttals for many of the reasons. Often times I have held my tongue, so as not to injure the precious fragile motivation the client brought to the initial meeting. I am sure many exercise professionals have thought the same things you are about to read in the next section, but have been reluctant to share.

Your Conscience

What if your conscience said things like those listed below? If some of this sounds sarcastic, that is because your conscience has no mercy and a real attitude. Your conscience is always present, whether you are listening or not.

You: I just don't have time today.
Conscience: *I hear this every day. If you would just stop whining about your schedule you would save at least 30 minutes a day.*

You: I don't have the money to join a gym.
Conscience: *Oh, I'm sorry, I didn't realize a gym was the only place you are allowed to exercise. I did not realize the city has tolls on the sidewalks. You have already paid your taxes for all the municipal parks, so take advantage if it.*

You: I don't have any place close enough.
Conscience: *So what you are saying is, that you don't have places closer than your living room to exercise in?*

You: I don't have any one to watch my child while I exercise.
Conscience: *I am assuming you choose not to go to a park or for a walk with your child. That would be too easy an answer. You know very well that you are not in a unique position. There are people out there saying the same thing waiting to meet you. You can become each other's solution while the other goes to exercise. If your gym does not provide child care, find another one. How many solutions do you need? What shade of green do you need the traffic light to be before you drive through the intersection?*

You: I am injured and can't do anything yet.
Conscience: *Oh, I am sorry, every tendon, ligament and muscle is just not up to the challenge today. Let's face it, you are not Evil Kanevil, having just broken 40 bones in a motorcycle jump gone wrong. You are just a person that has some tendonitis in your knee. If everything you could do with your leg hurts, do some upper body exercise for God's sake. There you go with the whining again. Stop already…*

You: My doctor has not cleared me to exercise yet.
Conscience: *You know darn well he said, "…No heavy lifting until we see how the MRI looks in two weeks." He did not say you could not walk, ride, hike or do calisthenics. Who are you trying to kid? Stop justifying your laziness.*

You: I don't know how to start. I am not sure what would be the best program for me.
Conscience: *If you were doing something, almost anything, it would be a better program than sitting there developing your remote control thumb. Look at that thumb; I think it is actually getting bigger. Don't get mired in the ideal program concept. You will get results from almost any program, with some honest effort.*

You: I need someone to workout with. I can't stay motivated.
Conscience: *You sure are motivated to shop endlessly without any moral support from you friends and family. If you have to find someone, hire a trainer. Talk to your friends whom already exercise or who have been thinking about starting. Why do you think there are so many books, magazines, exercise facilities and exercise equipment retailers? There are millions of people who think they should exercise on a regular basis, yet don't.*

You: After I lose some weight, I will get a membership to a gym.
Conscience: *My lord, do you hear yourself? You need to get into shape before you go to a place that will help you get into shape? That is like doing catalog shopping, so you have nicer clothes to wear when you go clothes shopping. Take your happy butt, fat or not, to the gym and get some work done.*

You: I want to get into shape, but exercise does not appeal to me.
Conscience: *…does not appeal to you? What kind of crap is that? You won't eat less, so your weight continues to increase. You have chosen a career that sits you in a chair all day. You have chosen to live in a condo, so you don't have*

yard work to do. I guess being 50 pounds overweight does appeal to you. At this point, walking from your car to your office is the most activity you get. The truth is that your lifestyle stinks, and all the money you make, and never have time to spend or are too tired to enjoy, is not worth it!

All is not lost. If you can face every day anew, not getting lost in yesterday's concerns, you can begin the journey toward a healthier happier life. Exercise to live; do not live to exercise.

Chapter 2

Finding The Motivation

How did you get here?

Motivation is a commodity not to be taken lightly. Motivation will come and go with the tides, Nil Desperandum—never despair.

"I have a terrible time getting started and an even tougher time maintaining the exercise program." What is your point? Everyone has that problem—just to different "degrees". The trick is to differ the "degrees" in the right direction. If we could stop talking about motivation and just get started, WOW, what a world it would be! This is not an attempt to belittle your feelings; rather, I want to show that the true obstacle is you. We are our own greatest enemies. We play mental games, volleying ideas, wrestling with pros and cons. Do I have time? Is this the best program for me? I don't want to hurt myself. Stop wondering what to do and do something, within reason. You can go for a 20 minute walk, for example. If you have done nothing but sit on the sofa or sit at your office desk for 15 years, don't go to the gym with your buddy and attempt everything he does. Most likely your friend has been exercising regularly for sometime, all the while asking you to come-along. You finally go, kill yourself, hurt for a week and swear you will never do that again. You have just given yourself the justification you have been looking for, not to exercise. Be realistic and respect your deconditioned state. It is real and your memories of what physical prowess you had in high school do not matter today.

You work 14 hours; yet want family time. Wrestle with your sons, swing your daughter, but do something. You just got back from flying 6 hours from South America, the jet lag is terrible, drown your pain in a nice swim or enjoy the ground beneath your feet on a walk. Do something!

A close friend said to me once, that she had hired a trainer to help her exercise. She was tired of the eight pounds she had gained and been unable to lose. I was floored by this, at first. This person worked for me for two years as a trainer and coach. She had gone through all the classes, certifications and professional tutelage to learn how to develop a comprehensive exercise plan. She knows what to do and has trained many people to get the exercise results they sought. She coaches high school athletes. You have to be good to motivate that group. Yet with all that, she could not motivate herself enough to do the exercise she wanted. I realize it was not the exercise she sought, but the potential results. The fact remained, her own knowledge and skill did not apply to her at this point. No one here is perfect. Even the pros need help sometimes.

The Big "C"

If you were fighting cancer, what would you do? If you were Clyde Grigsby (Unless you knew him, you would never have heard of him. He was a member of the facility I managed.) you would quietly never miss your exercise at the local YMCA. You would share a smile with the staff at the front desk, perhaps a kind word. You would proceed to the fitness center to do your usual routine. You would do what you could, depending on what your body would allow that day. You would never complain and always pleasantly greet your fellow exercisers. You would rarely ask for assistance and never be rude to someone while sharing equipment. If you were Clyde, you would happily donate to a worthy cause. All this you would do while never sharing your own pain from the cancer battle.

It was not until Clyde entered the hospital for the last time that I was told of his illness. He did not want to see anyone until he was stronger, which obviously never came to fruition. I was finally told one of the most powerful things I had ever been told. Clyde's son told us that Clyde suffered far more than he showed. On many days of his fight with cancer,

Clyde would get out of bed for one thing, the exercise session and fellowship at the YMCA. What kept him coming to exercise: the equipment, a warm smile from staff, the fellowship with other retirees, the spirited youngsters around the facility, the cancer fight? I am sorry to say that Clyde died before I took the time to get to know him better, and before he told anyone else what all his reasons were for staying active.

Motivated exercise is the blindingly brilliant key to successes in exercise, no matter your goals. Clyde had his. What is yours?????

One of the Luckiest Men

Motivation is developed in many ways from many experiences. Sometimes, it comes from experiences that simply give you a better perspective on life.

I was working with a great man once. Melber was 86 years of age and had never strength trained before, but was eager beyond compare. Melber turned out to be one of the luckiest men I have ever met. One day he showed up to train, wearing an old T-shirt. On the shirt was a picture of a WWII Intruder fighter plane. I asked him about the shirt. He perked-up and told me he use to fly one just like it, off an aircraft carrier during WWII. He proceeded to tell me he was the luckiest man he knew. My curiosity peaked; I welcomed his reason(s) why.

Once, while standing on the flight deck of the aircraft carrier, toward the end of the war, he saw an enemy plane diving right at the ship. The enemy Zero, dropped a bomb that headed directly at the deck, not far from Melber. As the bomb approached, Melber began to think the worst. As it got closer and closer, Melber froze—unable to run. The bomb slammed into the deck…bounced, not once, but twice, then went over the side coming to rest, in tact, on the bottom of the South Pacific. Melber was stunned. Simultaneously, with all his crewmates, Melber jumped for joy. The ship's crew theorized later that the firing pin of the bomb fell out during flight. Without the firing pin, the bomb became a dud!

Of the hundreds of people I have worked with, Melber had one of the best perspectives on things. He never really worried about what he could not change. He rarely expressed guilt for missing a workout, yet was dedicated. He knew his physical limitations and accepted them. His internal motivation came from his belief in God's gifts. If you believe God offers you life, then you know our role is to manage those assets well, including our bodies. Melber learned to appreciate his gifts everyday, never giving up the fight to live well and enjoy life.

As you have heard many times, we are all motivated by different things. When people would come to me and ask for an exercise program, one of the first things I would ask is, "Why are you here?" Most people are taken aback by the directness of the question. Many first reactions are negative, then, by my smile, they could see the playfulness of the approach. The idea is to keep the individual slightly off balance to provoke some sincere thought. Really, who am I to question someone's motives? Some trainers may be satisfied with collecting their money, not caring about why the person is there. Perhaps it is none of my business. I should just do my job, shut-up and keep the personal questions to myself. Many would agree with the idea of not getting too personal. I just cannot help wanting more information before I work with someone. My reason for inquiring was that I have grown tired of other peoples' failures to get the results they want because of a lack of commitment to the program they said they wanted. I am tired of the lip-service people give to motivation. I have watched too many people give too little sincere effort to programs I worked diligently to produce with them. I had developed an "Edge"—a real attitude. The "Edge", I like to call it, in this case, was my aggravation with failed efforts from people who thought this was the time for them to finally "Get Fit". I became so tired with unmotivated people, I would evaluate the person's motivation level, and if I saw a lack of sincerity, I would give the person to another trainer, or give them a simple down-and-dirty program that took little of my time. Was that the right thing to do? Of course not. Part of me, internalized the failures of some of my clients. I was tired of feeling like I had failed that person somehow. I wanted to work only with those who had the best chance to succeed, so I could live vicariously through their successes. The problem with success is that it too comes in many forms and varying degrees, often times unrecognized.

As time passed, I grew to see my calling differently. I began to take less personal stock in my client's success or failure. Giving people a fighting chance for success was how I defined my job. If they at least had the tools I helped provide, they might have a better chance to succeed when the right motivation came to them.

Adding regular exercise to your weekly routine is nothing short of a **lifestyle change**. If you think it is just a casual decision, you will never maintain a consistent exercise regime. If this concept is too harsh, so be it. The truth is that until reality is faced, you have a series of disappointing exercise experiences awaiting you.

What are the main reasons people start exercising? Over the years, I have challenged many people with this question. I have worked with all ages. Most often, people decide to "Get into Shape", "Get fit", "Loose Weight", "Trim Down", or "Bulk up" as the result of another lifestyle change or event.

John had just separated from his wife of 7 years, stopped drinking and wanted more from his career. A consistent exercise program, to get his body back into shape was the next step on his journey. He was going to stop worrying about those things and people he could not change. The only person he could change was himself. A change in our interpersonal relationships is one of the most common motives to begin exercise again. We all have been there, and understand the psychology. Some want to feel good and look good again. They find themselves "back on the market"— on the prowl (for the more aggressive people in the room). Perhaps the motives come from wanting to improve an existing relationship. Note this one obvious pitfall; do not do it for someone else. If you do, you will always be disappointed. Be reminded of the woman whose hateful spouse told her she was fat everyday of their marriage. Exercise and health was condemning—she would never look good enough. Similarly, there is the husband, being told he never takes care of himself, so often, he even hears it when no words are spoken. How many times can one hear, while looking at actors on TV, "If you looked more like that, I might sleep with you more often." Even said in jest, a portion of self-esteem dies. The strong person is going to take that and say, "I am happy with myself—I am secure." Most of us will find a reason not to even try, seeing too great a task. It is so true; we cannot rely on someone else for our motivation. Until you take control of your motivation you will be doomed to constant disappointment. A drill sergeant may be able to drive you through a workout, but you have to show up in the first place. For me, exercise was cathartic. Much of the tension of the day could be eased though tough physical exhaustion, like strength training. Exercise became my release valve. Those times in my life when I was exercising the least, I drank the most and was generally unhappy the most often. Strength Training offered me an emotional release. Have you ever noticed that when we feel like crap and act like it, we generally have poor interpersonal relations? Who wants to be with an emotional basket case? We all have to find the constructive ways of releasing our burdens that we can stick to. We are physical beings whose emotional strife is manifested into physical things. These things might be muscular tension, headaches or general feelings of malaise. Be aware of this when your burdens weigh heaviest.

Mary was a recently retired school principal, who found no time for exercise during her 30-year career. Now that she was retired, she thought she was going to have plenty of time to get into shape. Before I go any further, I must say that inactive retirement is practically an oxymoron. I have met many retirees in my career. Many have turned-out to be the busiest people I have ever met. I can't tell you how many people I have met who became busier once retired. It seems unrealistic that a very driven professional fades to inactivity once the "Gold Watch" is on. We are born with certain personality traits, exhibited throughout our lives in our work and leisure. To think those traits disappear because the job is not there, is nothing short of lying to ourselves. Later we will talk more about realistic exercise programming. For now but for now, suffice to say that changing your stripes is difficult, not impossible.

Many times, change is the result of a shift in priorities. Once I met a man who I just pegged wrong. His name was John. John was about 300 pounds, with about 120 of it being fat. John wanted to lose some weight, but more so, wanted to feel better. I am always happy to meet someone that I can help quickly. Many people do not realize that it takes very little activity to feel better—better about you, the world and even your life. Some might say that it is due to the endorphin release, or some other hormone. Whatever the reason, who cares why, if it will not hurt you and it works? Now, John had been exercising periodically for many years. Rarely did he ever feel like he was in a "routine". John had let everything else in his life control his schedule. I had to remind John that no one else was going to make time in his schedule for exercise but him. John obviously knew this bit of information. The only person he was leaving out of his schedule was himself. With that, John began his journey to a new lifestyle, to include exercise.

Needless to say that John's story ends very happily (Why else include it?). I saw John many months later. Through a strict exercise routine and some dietary changes, John had lost 60 pounds by the time I saw him. Even this far along on his journey to a healthier and happier lifestyle, John was far from done. His motivation and commitment had not peaked. He was changing mentally, physically and spiritually almost weekly. The enthusiasm and confidence he exuded was overwhelmingly infectious.

Successes in any exercise routine are infectious. Each goal that is achieved is like coal being thrown into the engine of a locomotive. The bigger the head of steam you can muster the loftier the goal achieved. To be sure, success is far from the only motivator to draw from.

As my own enthusiasm was fed by John, there are motivational triggers all around us. Perhaps the trick to exercise starting and adherence lies in recognizing the triggers, so they can be reproduced.

I would like to assume that you have identified your motivation, internalized it and can reproduce it. Now that you are ready, you need a path to follow. The path you should follow needs to be safe, first and foremost. Would you agree that an exercise plan that is detrimental to you health is not very healthy? Seriously, a well thought out plan considers many things. The place to start is with discussion of how you arrived at the physique you have today. What is your family's medical history? What is your personal medical history? What is your exercise history?

Chapter 3

Medical History/ Physical Constraints

Before designing an exercise program, we have to know where you are starting. Knowing your medical history is vital to creating a realistic and lasting program. What are the physical limitations? What are you capable of? What old or new injuries do you have that would make certain activities contraindicated (not indicated for use)? Has your doctor had that follow-up appointment with you to tell you results of the MRI you took? Do you suffer from diabetes, depression, heart problems, etc.?

There are many questions, such as these, which deserve consideration prior to starting a new exercise program. I will show you some examples of these questions. But, once the information is revealed, it may take the combined efforts of a trainer and a physician to prescribe a safe and effective program. Be honest and take this process seriously to avoid injury as a result of exercise that may be prescribed that may be contraindicated for you. I cannot tell you how many times I have pursued this process, and the person has given themselves a clean bill of health. Upon taking that person into the exercise room for the first workout, the truth comes out. Jim was a client that said he was fit as a fiddle. Once we began the initial cardiovascular session, Jim experienced shortness of breath and pain in his left knee. I stopped the session immediately and began asking questions…again.

Jim then recalled that he had knee surgery to remove cartilage about 10 years ago. He also had a number of experiences with shortness of breath.

He thought it just meant he was out of shape. I asked Jim to visit his doctor for further evaluation. It turned out Jim had a heart condition worth much attention. So, don't think it doesn't matter. If you are not an exercise professional, or physician, you may not be the best judge of the pertinence of a preexisting condition as it relates to the exercise prescription.

The following is an example of a questionnaire you might see as part of a quality exercise prescription. Some questionnaires may be far more or far less extensive. There are different theories as to how much information is necessary. The bottom line question is, "How, if at all, will my personal medical history affect my ability to do the exercise safely and effectively?" If you are not sure, ask the professionals.

Medical History Questionnaire

Last Name		*First Name*	*Middle initial*
Date of Birth	*Sex*	*Race*	*Home Phone*
Address		*City, State*	*Zip*
Work Phone		*Family Physician*	

Have you ever been diagnosed with any of the following:

- Diabetes   Yes   No
- Heart disease   Yes   No
- High Blood Pressure   Yes   No
- Migraines   Yes   No
- Cataracts   Yes   No
- Heart Murmur   Yes   No
- Angina   Yes   No
- Aneurysm   Yes   No
- High Cholesterol or triglycerides   Yes   No
- Stroke   Yes   No
- Thyroid problems   Yes   No

- Cancer   Yes   No
- Depression/nervousness   Yes   No
- Varicose Veins   Yes   No
- Gout   Yes   No
- Arthritis   Yes   No

- Do you ever experience any of the following:
- Shortness of breath   Yes   No
- Tingling or numbness in the extremities   Yes   No
- Swelling in the ankles or feet   Yes   No
- Leg pain or cramping   Yes   No
- Discomfort in the chest (heaviness/pressure)   Yes   No
- Uncontrollable coughing   Yes   No
- Extreme anxiety without apparent reason   Yes   No
- Skipped heartbeats or palpitations   Yes   No
- Dizziness   Yes   No

Personal History
    List any history of personal history of orthopedic injury to the back, neck, legs or arms.

Family History
    - Does anyone in your family have heart disease?   Yes   No
    - Does anyone in your family have a history of stoke? Yes   No
Medications
    List all medications you currently take or have been prescribed.

If you want the short version, many clubs use to evaluate new clients, it is called a

Physical Activity Readiness—Questionnaire (PAR-Q). Here is one example.

Yes No	1. Has your doctor ever said you have heart trouble?
Yes No	2. Do you frequently have pains in your heart and chest?
Yes No	3. Do you often have spells of severe dizziness?
Yes No	4. Has a doctor ever told you that you have a bone or joint problem, such as arthritis that has been aggravated by exercise, that might be made worse with exercise?
Yes No	5. Has your doctor ever said your blood pressure is too high?
Yes No	6. Is there a good physical reason not mentioned here why you should not follow an activity program if you want to?
Yes No	7. Are you over age 69 and not accustomed to vigorous exercise?

Source: Chisholm DM, et al. Physical Activity Readiness. BR Col Med J 17: 375-378, 1975.

With those questions answered, you have a much better idea about the issues that should be considered before a good exercise plan is designed and implemented.

Medications

Medications are a vital consideration when developing a program. Many people are unaware just how different medications can affect one's heart rate or metabolic rate.

For example, there is a category of heart medications called Beta-Blockers. This category of medications controls the heart rate, by keeping the heart rate down. In traditional programming for cardiovascular exercise, the trainer will suggest a heart rate range that should be maintained for optimal results. If the trainer prescribes a heart rate range of 130 to 140 beats per minute and the Beta-Blocker being taken keeps the heart rate below 100 beats per minute, you may over exert. In this case, you are at risk of injury in many ways. By knowing this, the trainer can suggest an alternative method of evaluating exertion. There is a method called RPE rating.

The RPE, or rate of perceived exertion, gives the exerciser a scale to rate your effort against how you feel.

Here is an example:

Rate	of Perceived Exertion (RPE)
6	
7	VERY, VERY LIGHT
8	
9	VERY LIGHT
10	
11	FAIRLY LIGHT
12	
13	SOMEWHAT HARD
14	
15	HARD
16	
17	VERY HARD
18	
19	VERY , VERY HARD
20	

Your doctor

I have some news for all of you outside the medical profession. Your doctor does not get paid to develop and evaluate your exercise program.

Doctors, generally, deal with problems not prevention. Many doctors will not consume themselves with your lifestyle if they do not have to. Most physicians have had little education in exercise physiology and biomechanics; however, it makes them no money to send you to a gym with an exercise plan. To be sure, there is definitely increased recognition and understanding of exercise benefits to health among the medical community. Please do not misunderstand the message being delivered. I am sure the vast majority of physicians care about their patient's health and well being. But, your doctor's basic job is not to teach you prevention and exercise; rather, it is to fix you when you are broken. The ideal situation exists when the doctor and exercise professional can share in the care and prevention of illness for a client. Here is the big rule when it comes to doctors and exercise professionals. If the doctor says not to do something, the exercise professional must abide by that recommendation when prescribing exercise. As an exercise professional, I am bound by the physician's recommendations, if they exist, about physical activity. I will not tell you to do anything that might be contradictory to the physician's orders. An important downfall to this ideal, is that some exercise advice from the medical community can come with no point of reference. I cannot tell you how many times I have had a new client in my office who was given a prescription by their doctor that limited the amount of activity the person did by saying, "Don't lift more than five pounds". What kind of useless advice is this? This person might lift more than five pounds just grocery shopping, working around the house or moving supplies at work. Why, all of a sudden, can't this person lift more than five pounds in a fitness center?

We can all appreciate the idea of playing it safe—being conservative. Usually, it is because it is better to be safe than sorry for the physician's insurance policy. The other reason may be that the physician has no real concept of this person's lifestyle demands and physical abilities. Once, I had a client who was one of the strongest women I have ever met. Shirley was in her mid-fifties, tall, slightly overweight and ready for anything. Shirley had received advice like that described above. After all the preliminary steps to prescribing exercise, it was time to evaluate her capability. We tested her on several items of strength training equipment before getting to the Shoulder Press machine. For those who are not familiar with this machine, you sit with a long pad to support your back. You have two handles on either side of your head. You take each handle and press them over your head. Notoriously, women lift far less weight than men on this exercise. There are anatomical, physiological, and sociological reasons that may answer why. That was not important. This woman pressed as much weight overhead as any man could in a similar situation. She far outshined her female counterparts. It turned out that Shirley grew-up stacking bails of hay with her brothers on the family farm. This woman would only have gotten weaker, limiting herself to lifting 5 pounds.

This brings me to the next point. Often times, advice from physicians, about exercise, can be vague. Is the 5 pounds free weight or is that machine weight? Even I paid attention in 8th grade class long enough to know that once you employ the use of pulleys, you alter the work being done. If the weight is guided by something like steel rods, in the case of exercise machines, it further changes the dynamics of the weight being lifted.

Often times the best program comes from trial and error. There are too many variables that are not considered when vague exercise advice is given.

Finding Your Baseline

One of the first things I do with a new client is ask them if I can take their heart rate and blood pressure. With these two items of information I can begin to evaluate a baseline. "Why does it matter?" you may ask. Most people do not know what their true resting heart rate is. If you take your heart rate first thing in the morning, after putting your feet on the floor right out of bed, you may come close to a resting heart rate. How can a trainer use this information?

The trainer can use your resting heart rate information to determine a cardiovascular exercise prescription. For example, part of the exercise prescription might say that you should do 20 minutes of cycling at 60% of your maximum heart rate level using the Karvonen formula (ref.: Astrand, P. O., and K. Rodahl. Textbook of work physiology, 2nd ed., New York: McGraw-Hill, 1977. Karvonan, M.J., E. Kentala, and O. Mustala. The effects of training on heart rate. A longitudinal study. Annales Medicinae Experimentalis et Biologiae Fenniae, 1957, 35:305-315. The formula looks like this:

Heart Rate During Exercise=
Heart Rate while resting +0.60[Maximum Heart Rate{220—age x
(.6 to .8)}—Heart Rate while resting]

The idea is that we can more accurately prescribe exercise if we consider the individual's baseline fitness level. What could happen is that you generally have a higher than average resting heart rate. If your doctor has told you that there is no problem related to this higher than average HR, then we can prescribe a more intense program. That is, if you are prescribed exercise that is too low in intensity, your results will be hampered. For example, if your average resting heart rate is 90 bpm, then using the formula above, you have to keep a higher heart rate to exercise at the same rate of perceived exertion, as someone with a resting heart rate of 75 bpm.

I was sent an e-mail some time ago, entitled, "The Interview". To paraphrase, an individual dreams he or she has an interview with god. The individual asks God, "What surprises you most about mankind?" God answered with several things, but there was one that caught my attention most. In this email God says, "That they lose their health to make money and lose their money to restore their health." I have seen this truth lived out so many times, I stopped counting. If we do not learn from the mistakes of others, therein lays a tragedy. If we do not learn the lessons available to us from our mistakes and successes, it is just plain stupidity. Learn from your mistakes and change for success where failure was present before. The next step to developing a quality exercise program is evaluating what you have done in the past.

(With tangible personal limits in mind, it is time to consider the next limit to regular exercise.)

Chapter 4

Exercise History

During this part of the information gathering, the client is to be honest. Not honest with the Exercise Professional, but most honest with themselves. A simple question such as, "How often do you exercise?" might turn into a dissertation of high school athleticism. The proper response from the trainer is, "…, but you are 45 years old now. What have you done lately?" You say, "Oh, well, I have a very active job. I'm on my feet all day." "Then why do you think you need an exercise program designed for you?" I say. "My doctor told me that I need to lose weight", you say. I say, "If your job is so active, why are you 40 pounds overweight?" Either you define "active" differently than most, or you simply eat enough for two.

The body becomes accustomed to whatever you do consistently—work is a perfect example. Just because you are a mason who lifts bricks and cinder blocks all day, does not mean you will have a bodybuilder's physique. The body only works as hard as is required to accomplish the work (muscle recruitment). The body does not maintain muscle mass it does not use. No, you cannot "will" your body to be stronger; although, many have tried. Imagine your actions are the teacher, while your body is the student. When you exercise you teach your body what you want it to do. You teach it how much you want to lift and what intensity you want it to achieve. Unlike a five year old child, your body listens to the challenges you give it. It responds by adapting to the workload. The body, as a machine, is a marvel of adaptation.

If you do not feed the machine the right data (physical challenge) it will not adapt correctly.

The issue lies in what you have done for your body lately. What are your exercise successes (i.e. weight loss, muscle gain, shape change, etc.)? How often did you exercise? What exercises did you choose?

Here is a positive note: It is easier to reacquire a previous level of physical fitness than to get there originally. If your body was once accustomed to running 5 miles 3 or 4 days per week, it will be easier to get back to that level. The body will retain some of the physiological adaptation needed to accomplish the task. Think of riding a bike, you never forget how. The body will retain some of the development of the nervous and circulatory pathways required to ride the bike, no matter how long it has been. Of course, I have seen many adults try to reacquire their youthful cycling spirit and crash miserably. But, luckily, pride was usually the only thing hurt. They could still ride, but it may take some time before they are proficient again.

Psychologically, you have fewer barriers, because you remember accomplishing the task before. When we know we have accomplished something before, we are more easily driven to that end. When trying to bench press 200 pounds, for the first time, there is a great deal of self-doubt. These doubts can sometimes be our greatest obstacles.

Back to reality, those of us beyond our teen years must remind ourselves of this, and act our ages. I am not saying we need to be scared of the exercise, or that we are too old. To the contrary, I believe in life-long exercise. So as not to be foolish, we need to quickly find our new limits, by listening to our bodies. Some people walk onto the basketball court and feel that youthful exhilaration again. This feeling can be hazardous to your health. You may find yourself quickly dragging—"sucking-wind", missing all your shots, and having to rest after every point. Reality can be a cruel mistress, hard on the body and detrimental to motivation. After the body stops regular activity, research shows a potential loss in muscle mass, up to 7% every 10 years after age 30. Doing the math, at age 45, with 15 years of inactivity, you may have a loss in musculature of 10.5%. WOW! I know that thought hurts. Keep in mind, this is different for everyone depending on disease, physiology, lifestyle, diet and exercise history. There are those who were very out-of-shape in high school. Yet, later in life, those same people discovered a very healthy and active lifestyle. Now they find themselves in better condition many years beyond high school.

Always attempting to move forward, let us leave the past where it belongs—in the past. All the past is worth is education, whether that past be positive or negative. From our personal history's with exercise, we need to divine personal patterns and physical limits. If you are to design a program for yourself, you must start slowly to avoid all the pitfalls which are detrimental to your motivation.

Chapter 5

What You Like To Do

What are you willing to do?

After we go though all the different activities you have tried in the past, we should be able to find something you will be willing to do. Once, I was asked to design a program for a young man whose only goal was to look better on the beach, (Who doesn't?).

He and I were at the program design phase where we narrow down the things he is accustomed to doing or willing to do. We began listing exercises.

Me: "Do you like cycling?"

Him: "No."

Me: "…How about jogging?"

Him: "No, not really."

Me: "How do you feel about aerobics?"

Him: "No, no rhythm…"

Me: "Do you like circuit training?"

Him: "No. I'm not into that."

Me: "Do you prefer using free weights?"

Him: "No, can't say that I do."

Me: "Ok, it sounds like I can't help you. What if I asked, what you are willing to do?"

Him: "Oh, well, I'm willing to do all those things."

Me: "Now we are getting somewhere."

The moral of the story is, sometimes, it is not a matter of what the person likes to do, but a matter of what the person is willing to do to achieve their goals. It is important to qualify the concept of what someone is willing to do to achieve goals. When I refer to a willingness to do certain things, that does not include radical diets, extreme sports, plastic surgery, illegal steroid use, etc. A willingness to do what it takes refers to practicing proven safe methods for activity that can burn calories and effectively improve physical strength.

When choosing activities to use in a regular exercise program, it helps to start with those the body is already use to. Almost all of us have to walk to get from place to place, through our homes, to our cars and around stores. Since the body has already developed the nervous and circulatory pathways to walk, somewhat efficiently, it is an easy place to start. Alternatively, if you choose swimming as your cardiovascular activity, but have not been in the pool for 10 years, you may have some difficulty. The body develops its circulatory system and nervous system, and muscular system to handle the tasks it is asked to do **on a regular basis**. If you have not asked your body to swim on a regular basis it cannot be ready to.

Finally, now that you know what you are willing to do, what are you going to do? What result comes of a disappointing experience? Most likely, you experience a feeling of failure. But like anything, if swimming is what you choose to do, and you have not been swimming regularly, it will just take longer before the activity is comfortable. Now that you know what you are going to do, it is time to set some goals.

Chapter 6

Realistic Goal Setting

I cannot tell you how often I've been told, "I have my work in order, I have my personal life right, I am ready to jump-in and do 5 days a week, 2 hours a day." My response is, "Are you crazy? How much pain do you want to suffer through?" This I say on the inside. Very few people want to hear the truth. Most people do not want to hear, "You have done no regular physical activity for 10 years and you want to jump-in?" The truth is, as I have said before, if you have not been active, this new regime is nothing short of a **lifestyle change**. If you believe any less, you will fail to reach these vary lofty goals. Any goal we set which requires action that is divergent from anything you presently do, needs to be tempered with realism.

Now that you are depressed, discouraged, and annoyed with me, let us face facts. If you are a workaholic, alcoholic, or similar, you are probably obsessive. This means, you can easily burn-out on this new lifestyle if you approach it too aggressively. If you tend to melt into the sofa every night, what charm, what invitation would a thinly padded exercise cycle seat hold for you? Set goals that are tempered by a realistic plan are usually achievable. It is the rare individual who makes any changes cold turkey. You might say, "I have done it before." Perhaps you have, but at what age and fitness level? True, the body is a marvel of adaptation, changing to meet new demands placed upon it. However, when those challenges are too great, the body breaks-down, and recovery can be painful and devastating to motivation. Who hasn't approached a daunting task with starry-eyed enthusiasm, only to fall flat as a pancake?

Avoid such pitfalls by doing what you know you can, then building on it. Do you know you can walk around the block? Do you know you can lift 100 pounds? As a trainer, one of my roles is to evaluate your current fitness level and temper your goals, as I did with John.

John had not exercised regularly for 10 years. He was devoted to work and family equally. John usually ate well—healthfully, but never made time for his own physical activity. When John came to me, his kids were in high school-wanting nothing to do with Dad. His wife was very socially active. John finally had time for John—himself. After evaluating his level of conditioning, I was not surprised to hear John tell me he was ready for a program consisting of 5 days a week for no less than one hour a day. I told John, that although that sounded great, perhaps that was not the ideal plan just yet. Then I said, "Now tell me what is realistic." At this moment, John, as so many others, had to pause. Sure, John had the time to put into an aggressive program; more importantly, did he have the motivation and commitment? Was he being honest with himself? John spoke again, "I guess if I was to be realistic, I might spend 30 minutes 3 days a week." I thanked John for answering correctly—because that is what I was going to suggest. John took the next great step in planning his program.

We now had a realistic framework with which to fill appropriate exercises he was willing and wanting to do.

I want to close this section with the toughest issues I face as a strength and conditioning professional. I entered the exercise science field, because I enjoy seeing people improve themselves—have successes. Some may say I am in the field because all trainers have a sadistic side. Torturing people is only part of the enjoyment. I am kidding…for the most part. As a trainer, I had to be realistic with how much help I could offer people. When you want to help someone in failing health, how do you do it? In some of my earlier experiences with people having serious and lasting health problems, I found a great sense of failure. I did not want to face the reality of deteriorating health in some of my clients. When you train people regularly, you get to know them. You can even form lasting friendships. Sometimes I grasped their enthusiasm for the potential help I could provide, no matter the reality. One such client was Bubba.

Bubba, at 85 years of age, and his doctors, wanted him to get some activity. Bubba suffered from a heart that no longer pumped so good (congestive heart failure), permanent muscle contractions (contractures) and a host of other problems. After evaluating his situation, with the aid of his physician, we set some goals such as:

- to be able to stand-up from a chair after 6 sessions
- to be able to walk for 5 minutes without stopping in 2 weeks

As you can imagine, goals like those for Bubba would not be lofty aspirations for the average person. For Bubba, these goals proved very challenging. At first, Bubba showed modest progress. I would go to his condo for 30 minutes 3 days a week. I wanted to help Bubba, perhaps more than he could be helped. All too quickly, I could see Bubba had good days and bad days. We all have good and bad days, but his were more obvious. After just one month Bubba began to cancel one or two times per week. We both realized that his physical limits were frustrating him. He even had a sense of failing me, in my efforts. I did not want to believe that we were doing all he was capable of. He looked for me to be his cheerleader, saying "Get up, let's go." However, I was dying on the inside, becoming frustrated for him. I could see his disappointment, no matter how hard he tried. For a trainer, a self-motivated client is more rare than common. Many people give lip service to wanting results, while showing minimal effort. In exercise, success and feeling better are the greatest motivators. Bubba was experiencing neither. His doctor, Bubba, nor I could reverse the course of his failing health. After just 2 months, Bubba and I stopped working together. He had a series of hospital stays that left him in an indigent care situation. His doctor's efforts could only be focused on minimizing Bubba's pain, at best. Later that year, Bubba died. As a trainer, even knowing the reality, was not enough to save me from feeling I had failed him somehow.

Bubba's situation serves as an extreme case for most people in my profession. People who do physical therapy and indigent care see Bubba's situation far more often. Having spoken to many physical therapists and physicians, even knowing life's cruel side, does not make it easier to face. We must approach a program with reality in mind, building on successes. We need to continually reevaluate our goals, less we stagnate.

The chapters in this book are organized as a series of questions. Here is a summary of some important questions you need to ask yourself when establishing goals for your new exercise program. These questions are presented as though the person is not in a consistent exercise program.

1. Why do you want to begin exercising now?
2. What are your top three motivators to beginning a program at this time?
3. What are your physical constraints?
4. What activity is your body most used to?
5. What are your exercises of choice?
6. What equipment do you have available to you?
7. Will you have a partner?
8. How much time, weekly, are you going to plan for this program?
9. Is there a time limit set for this goal? (i.e. a pending wedding)
10. On a scale of 1 to 5, 5 being the highest priority, what priority are you going to give your exercise-related goals?

Chapter 7

Exercise Plan

We have spent much time gathering information to support a realistic plan for a successful exercise experience. You have the motivation. You know your proper health limitations. You know what you are willing to do, and you know your goals.

The exercise plan/program is the last step before beginning. Before we get to that, how do we fit the lifestyle you have now with the new one that includes the exercise plan?

Which days of the week will we apply the prescription to? What time of day works best for you? Are you a morning person or a night owl? Will you prioritize the workout in you day so you do it first? Will you spend the entire day trying to find time to fit it in? How much time will your exercise get in your busy week? Let us look at which days work best for you.

Which days

Even this simple question has shown to be too cumbersome for some to negotiate. Again, it is about being absolutely honest with yourself. If you are going to exercise 3 days per week, does Monday, Wednesday, and Friday work best? Keep in mind that a plan that includes less than 3 days per week is barely a maintenance program; however it is still something to build on. If you like to celebrate the end of the week with your friends on Friday night, will you really go to the gym after work? Be careful to strive for balance when choosing exercise over entertainment or fellowship and vice versa. You may find yourself resenting it later. It is the same thing as

34

depriving yourself of cake while on a diet. After a while of craving the cake, while denying yourself the cake, you create an uncontrollable desire. Most people will find that they binge on the things they have deprived themselves of when they go off the diet. Moderation is key. A famous French queen said, "Let them eat cake". What she should have said was, " Let them eat cake in moderation." If the queen had today's information, I am sure she would have modified her infamous statement. I heard she was a reader. That aside, if at times you cut a workout short to meet some friends or change days, it is not the end of your "hot streak". You are not a bad person and you should not let it affect your motivation.

With that, it is time to look at some exercise prescriptions that have worked for others. Perhaps one of them, or a modified version, will work for you.

Time of Day

While you stay motivated, get serious about time. If you treat your exercise time with priority, you will fit it into your day. If you "play it by ear" and hope to "squeeze it in" at some point in the day, you will fail. If you enter your exercise session in your journal, type it, touch it, write it, you raise the chance of success.

Plans

Let us look at some beginning plans that have been successful for others. The workouts that follow are based on the idea of having access to a full fitness center. Later in this section we will talk about workouts at home with limited equipment availability. The program below is an example. **There are detailed programs listed in the appendix.**

....

Program #1

3 Days per week (M, W, F)—35 to 40 minutes

Warm-up

Light Stretch

Cardiovascular—15 minutes stationary cycling or walking—60% MHR
Cool-down—no less than 5 min.
Strength Training—20 minutes

- Leg Press
- Leg Extension
- Leg Curl
- Pull-down
- Chest Press
- Chest Fly
- Shoulder Press
- Triceps Extension
- Biceps Curl
- Abdominal Curl

Choosing the Initial Starting Points

For strength training, when choosing the initial weights, be conservative and BE CONSERVATIVE. Your first attempt should be easy. "But Why?" you shriek. "I want results, I want to feel like I have done something." I appreciate your enthusiasm, but I want you to comeback and see me for the next workout. In my early days as a trainer, I would have put you through your paces from day one. I would assume everyone wanted the same intensity in his or her workouts as I had in mine. I soon learned it was taking people a week or more to come back to the fitness center and sometimes, did not see them again. A few people actually became ill in the middle of the workout and had to run to the restroom. I was naive enough to believe that they must have been getting a cold or the flu. However, the trend was undeniable. These people had come in feeling fine. Some had eaten, some had not. The common threads were a new intense exercise program and a deconditioned person. I realized the trainer—me, needed to keep his own enthusiasm in check. Since you are working to be your own trainer, this means you.

So, what should that first workout feel like?

- **You should feel the muscle working, but not to fatigue.**

There will be plenty of time for high intensity exercise sessions, later. The first workout is actually part of the information gathering we have been doing up to now.

During the first workout you are telling your body what you will be doing to it. Again, be kind to this body as it is the only one you have. On the other hand, the human body is a marvel of adaptation. From the first lift of the barbell, the first 5 minutes of jogging, your body says, "Whoa! What is going on? This feels very different. I need to make some changes." Your body starts to immediately make adjustments—physiological adaptations. The body is constantly trying to maintain balance (equilibrium) in its chemical levels. The body wants to better handle the load the next time it is faced with the challenge, be it lifting a weight or running some distance. If you have not heard of the term "progressive resistance", listen-up. Without progressive resistance, we cannot improve.

Progressive resistance is how we improve and grow. Without an ever-increasing challenge, the body has no new challenge to ADAPT to. How many of us have used the same weights, the same running distance, same intensity for countless workouts, and when it's done, wondered, "Why am I not progressing?" While I was working for a club in Virginia, a member came to me and asked me why he was no longer seeing progress. He told me he runs 5 days per week, 5 miles a day. He had been doing this for 10 years. After I applauded his consistency, I asked him when he last felt he was seeing results. He said, it had been about 9 years. I asked him if he ever changed his intensity, speed, or distance. He inquisitively told me no. I said, "Well, what you've got here is one hell of a consistent maintenance program. In an exercise program, as in any endeavor, you will improve, stay the same, or decline. Improving—progressing, will be driven by an effort the body has to improve upon. If you don't increase the weight lifted, reps done, distance, speed, resistance, or time there is no new challenge for the body to adapt to. With that, lets talk more about the initial workout.

The first workout is meant to find a baseline, a starting point. In the initial sessions we found a baseline heart rate. We have to know where our strength levels are. All progress is based on where we start during that first workout. If you try too much, too soon, you are not giving your body time to adapt to the new physical demands. A part of the physiological adaptation process is training the body to recover in a reasonable amount of time. The body actually does not improve during the exercise sessions. It improves during the time you rest. **STOP right there!** I know what you are thinking. By what I just said you may have been estimating that you have not been out of exercise, you have been resting from your last workout for the last 10 years. There is such a thing as too much rest. Generally, the research shows that an adequate recovery from cardiovascular sessions is 24 hours, while higher intensity exercises, such as strength training, take about 48 hours. These times will vary among individuals. Also, plan on a longer recovery period after your first several workouts. Better to be safe than sorry. Listen to your body. If it is still very sore, it may need another day to recover.

Chapter 8

Nutrition—Calories In-Kilocalories Out

It is the simplest of notions, yet one of the most overdone topics in this country today.

How many times have you heard or read about the latest and greatest diet? How many diets have you tried? Why can't you seem to find the formula, when you have tried so many? I am here to tell you, for the vast majority of us, that the formula is as easy as you make it. Don't waste your time searching for a different formula, when the best formula has been with you since you were a child. Follow the four food groups. Eat less. The fastest way to trim unwanted calories from your day is to not consume them in the first place. This is the part where most people say things like, "Easy for you to say. I have no will-power." Or perhaps you say, "I like eating. I enjoy food." Fine, enjoy food. No one is saying you cannot eat. The excessive consumption of food is killing this country. As the portions served in restaurants have grown, so has this county's collective waistline. Wait just a moment. This is not a cry to blame the restaurants. Overeating occurs at home, at the family barbecue, in schools…anywhere we want. Nor should we starve. Enjoy what you want; just eat less of it. There is no one who can save you from yourself…for long. Take control of your habits, both good and bad. Who loves you more than you? If you answer that question with the name of someone other than yourself, you have other issues to deal with. In the event you do not know what that help is, ask a professional to help with the discovery process. Once you see the issues, you can begin to take action to positively change your eating habits.

Kilocalories vs. calories

Earlier I told you that the fastest way to trim unwanted calories from your day, is to not consume them at all. Do you realize that the large, very greasy hamburger, you had for lunch will roughly take an hour of hard running to burn-off? Let us assume this burger meal is the one that is continually putting you over the top—over what your body needs to maintain its weight.

Since most people tend to eat in similar patterns each day, yet only exercise periodically, in a week's time you may have **overeaten** to the tune of 3200 calories, or almost one pound. If you follow the same pattern for 1 year, you will have overeaten more than 166,000 calories, or 47 pounds. It is that simple to over eat. The commitment and dedication to remove the unwanted pounds is a far greater struggle. Again, no one said not to **ever** eat the burger, simply eat fewer of them. As you stare at the unfinished food on your plate, ask yourself, "What is more important to me, losing the unwanted pounds or wasting food?" If you feel that badly about wasting food, take all the cans and dry goods you have sitting in your pantry to a shelter. That group rarely over eats. It is not an option for them. I say this, not to be crass, rather to remind us of all that we have. **Gluttony, usually, only serves one.**

Well-rounded no more

If you can't seem to eat from the four food groups, try to round out your diet with a multivitamin. **Why?** Most professionals are struggling with the concept of suggesting supplements. The reason is that most people could get all the vitamins and minerals they need daily, if they would just eat a well-rounded diet. However, the fact remains, that the majority of us rely on restaurants and cafeterias to supply, at least a portion of, our daily dietary consumption. These places are in the business of making food taste good so they can sell more and more of it. At least many eateries try to make the food taste good. Are we to blame the restaurants and cafeterias for our overeating or poor food choices? Certainly not! Most eating establishments have the well-rounded meals available. We have to get better at recognizing appropriate portion sizes, and at seeking the heart healthy items on the menu. Remember, that if your diet is not as balanced at it should be, it may benefit you to take a multivitamin. I am not a fan of taking megadoses of specific vitamins. Most of the time vitamins and minerals need to be consumed together so they can interact and be used effectively in the body. Always consult your physician before trying any new supplements.

Since supplements are such a hot topic today, we must remember there is something called an RDA (Recommended Daily Allowance) that tells us how much of the vitamins and minerals we need. Food manufacturers and processors are publishing a wealth of information on food labels these days. If you have not read a food label lately, you may find it very telling. After reading your labels and be sure you try to take any vitamin, or like supplement, with food. Your body will have a better chance of absorbing the nutrients when in the presence of digestive enzymes being used to breakdown the solid food having been consumed.

I feel compelled to quickly address the issue of appetite suppressants. Appetite suppressants and extreme diets come with some risk and, usually, some side effects.

First, remember that your goal is never simply to lose the weight, but to keep it off.

Appetite suppressants and extreme diets are like the substitute teacher in school, who you liked for giving you the answers on quizzes, but rarely learned anything from. The teacher who challenged you to study and discover things for yourself is most likely the teacher who taught you the most. Appetite suppressants and extreme diets give temporary relief to a lifelong struggle. If you do not practice self-control, appropriate eating habits, and discipline, why would you magically acquire it once you have lost the weight? To be sure, miracles do happen in dieting, but let us assume the Lord is saving miracles for bigger things. If over eating is a problem you would like to change, you must discover, uncover and practice. Discover how many calories is too many for you. Uncover new ways to eat less. Practice the discipline that you uncover. There are many resources available to help you on your dietary journey.

I have a great web page for you, *www.health.gov*. Checkout what the Surgeon General is telling the country. It is pretty good stuff. You will find many answers.

Chapter 9

My Home Gym

My home gym, currently, is composed of a jump rope, the floor and the street outside. Hershel Walker, former professional football player, serves as a wonderful example to a simple exercise plan resulting in fantastic conditioning. Hershel has told the story many times of how he received some simple advice to improve his physique. It turned out that Hershel's sister used to always beat him in footraces. The local high school football coach told him that if you wanted to run faster, then run. If you want to get stronger, do push-ups and pull-ups. Hershel took the coach's advice. As I understand the story, he was beating his sister within 6 months, never losing a race to her again. As his athleticism grew, so did his physique. Even as his football and track careers blossomed through college, he never touched any free weights; and yet, he was heralded as one of the best-conditioned athletes in the world. I know it sounds simple, but so can be a successful exercise program. It can also be as complicated as you make it.

The search for the perfect home gym-complement of equipment can be mind-bending if you look at all the different things available. I used to have a bench and 300 pounds of Olympic free weights, hand weights, a curl bar, ankle weights, a pull-up bar, etc.. Thanks to my divorce, I have the home gym I described in the first sentence of the chapter. I can hear my ex-wife now, "You know well that you did not use that stuff very much. You also decided to donate the equipment to YMCA." She was right about that. Even an avid exerciser may not use all the things at his disposal all the time. I much preferred going to the fitness center, anyway. I found too many distractions at home. If you can work past distractions

43

at home, consider forming a home gym with all you have at your access. Distractions aside, how do you discover a good mix of equipment for you?

Review the Programming Steps

After you have gone through the major steps in developing a program, then search for the right equipment. For example, if you like bike riding, get a bike, etc..

What have you tried?

If you have never tried the equipment you want to buy, you are potentially making a big mistake. Have you, yourself, or know someone who has purchased equipment that is now collecting dust somewhere in a house? We are geared to believe the infomercials and "BUY NOW". Why?…because advertising works. Just because advertising works, does not mean the equipment works for you. Remember, we do not buy out of need, as much as we buy out of want. We want to buy. We want results; however, we want it to be easy, comfortable and immediate.

There are hundreds of different pieces of exercise equipment on the market that have found homes in which they have been cherished, almost worshiped. This worship comes in the form of minimal use so the piece will maintain its "like new" appearance and function. Please do not miss the sarcasm here.

There is an exercise piece on the market today that had a brilliant advertising campaign. The company sold thousands and thousands of their devices. But, when many people got them home, they realized it was not nearly as easy to operate. The person on TV looked so graceful; it almost looked effortless. While, simultaneously, the person on TV was burning twice as many calories as walking could burn. In several of the facilities I worked in over the years, I used to teach people how to use the machine. Out of every 10 people I showed the exercise piece to, 5 could not do it and 3 of the five that could do it, did not enjoy it. This is a common problem.

So try the device first, making sure it is something you will use. My mother usually did not try out the equipment first.

I love my mother very much, but the things she has purchased without ever trying them, would boggle your mind. From treadmills, to ski machines, to abdominal rockers, to elastic bands and benches, she keeps trying the latest and greatest waiting to find something that will keep her interest. It is not that she is an easily distracted woman, but she really is. What I find very interesting, is that she is now exercising regularly. She is in a traditional fitness center setting and she walks. She has lost 30 lbs. and her asthma is in-check. Certainly the routine is not the latest and greatest, but definitely successful.

Be smart with your money and your exercise.

What to look for

You are an intelligent person, who has a good idea of what you might want in a piece of exercise equipment. However, you may want a little help in deciphering all the information there is today about exercise and the exercise equipment. The first thing is to remember that no matter how efficient the device is at helping burning calories, you still have to use it! The real point is not to belittle, but to create a sense of realism. So many people have asked me, "What is the best exercise"? My immediate response is, " The one you will do everyday." Again, it is not a matter of need to do, should do, but want to do. You might be saying to yourself, "I don't want to exercise; I have to." Let's not get mired in semantics. You did it, or are doing it, because you chose and continue to choose to do it. You either chose to exercise, or you chose to sit on the sofa all day and watch TV. Now, those who do not add unwanted pounds, while using "sofa sitting" as their only activity, have discovered how to eat appropriately to their activity level, or should I say lack of activity level? The bad news is that they are losing muscle, which lowers overall metabolism over time.

Since time is usually of the essence, let us begin to determine some smart exercise equipment purchases. As with any purchase, you should identify several categories and apply a high and low rating to them. Here is an example of how you might begin to rate a particular item. Ask the sales representative about a "Good, Average, or Poor" rating in these categories: Durability, Adjustability, Service Warranty and Repair History.

Durability is a very important category, because you may be comparing a home model to a commercial model. Using treadmills as an example in this discussion, there are many models of treadmill on the market today, ranging from self-propelled units to underwater treadmills that cost more than $10,000. Always remember that the average person is not going to want to invest the money it takes to have a commercial treadmill in their home. Can it be a good investment? Yes, the higher price usually means the treadmill has a greater degree of durability. It is made of superior material, handles more weight, the motor is larger, and has greater programmability. Additionally, the commercial systems often have longer and wider belts with better warranties. If you decide you want to have a treadmill for your home, it will most likely have to be smaller than a commercial unit, lighter and come with few options. I am not saying you won't like the home model treadmills. The fact remains that you will usually notice the different feel between the home and commercial models. That difference is much like that between the feel of driving a large four-door car and a small two door coupe.

Watch the mark-up

As in any industry, the exercise equipment market has its honest and less than honest vendors. Also, like any larger purchase, you should listen to your friends and get some additional referrals.

I am aware of a few companies that even receive awards for maintaining higher mark-ups. The manufacturers will also give plenty of bonus or incentive to the retailer for the higher markups. Of course this is nothing new, but some people tend to forget the rules of smart shopping when they look at exercise equipment. I might assume that it is due to the perceived "foreign territory". People new to exercise think they need to be told everything. Here is a good rule: If the retailer spends more time telling you what to buy than asking you what you want the piece for, they are selling you what they want to sell you, not necessarily which piece is better for you.

Check the second hand market

Why is there such a growing second hand market for exercise equipment? It is evident in the number of second hand retail stores that have emerged over the last ten years. Perhaps it is due to the fact that there is so much home equipment that is not getting worn- out. Rather, much home exercise equipment is just collecting dust. Dust just does not wear out equipment like actual use does. So, you end up with a lot of equipment almost as good as new, being resold in the second exercise equipment market. Even some retailers will refurbish equipment and put it back on the floor for sale. Be sure to check the warranty that may be available on the refurbished equipment you are considering buying.

Finally, the proper use of almost any piece of exercise equipment can help you attain results. Without a doubt, some pieces are definitely better than others. It is the application of said equipment where most people can falter. Be sure, you follow all manufacturers' advice.

Years ago, I was approached by a neighbor about accepting a gift of a piece of exercise equipment he did not want any longer. It was a type of inversion equipment. At the advice of a physician, this neighbor's wife was given the suggestion of using the device to help her stretch her spine and strengthen her abdominal muscles. For those not familiar with the device, it was a platform (like a cot) with gravity boots attached. The platform was attached to a hinged rack. Once you stepped into it, and fastened the boots to the ankles, you could rock back like a seesaw. You were to rock over to an inverted position, hanging by your feet. The inverted position allowed the user to relieve pressure on the spine and perform abdominal exercises. If the user's abdominal were too weak to sit up, the user could adjust the distance of the rear motion so they did not rock back too far.

To make a long story short, the neighbor's wife tried to use the device while no one else was home. She had gotten stuck in the inverted position. By the time the husband had returned, the wife was screaming bloody murder to be helped out of the device. She never used it again. Being the young exercise enthusiast, I took the device and put it to use. The first time I used it I could understand how she had faltered in her use of the device. This is easily not a recommended device for many people by today's standards. I felt guilty for laughing at the image of this poor woman trapped in this device that was designed to help her ailing back. I also saw the opportunity for serious injury.

Choose your exercise equipment wisely.

Spotters and Partners

Just because you are at home does not mean you may not need help. Be careful not to test strength limits while alone. Stay within known physical limits while exercising alone. Any levels of progression should be subtle and attainable. Protect yourself by finding a partner whenever possible.

Chapter 10

Exercise Myths

Why do they still believe?

Why is it, no matter how often or by which expert, exercise myths are rebuked, we keep finding believers of the lies? Let's get this out of the way. There is no such thing as spot reducing, magic pills, fat reducing ointments, etc.! There, I said it—I feel better. Our bodies are made to function in certain ways. Rely on the most perfect machine in the world to function. When we alter function, we end up with side effects, usually negative ones. Sometimes our bodies need help—the human machine malfunctions. Even the things we use to help can alter function. The body is always trying to maintain balance—metabolic physiologic equilibrium, just as the balance of spirit, mind and body is continually pursued.

Undeniable Facts

Fat does not burn fat! Muscle burns fat! Fat is a storage item. Muscle is an active tissue requiring energy. A simple explanation of fat burning implies that fat burns in a physiological flame of carbohydrate. The University of Massachusetts in Boston (Research Quarterly for Exercise and Sport, Vol. 70, No. 2, pp.150-156), reported that men who are muscular have more calorie-burning power during aerobic exercise than less muscular men of the same weight, according to a recent study. If you take stock in these findings, our goal is to add muscle which will, in turn, burn more fat.

Why not try the magic weight loss pill

All too often we have seen so clearly the risks, ramifications, side effects and health hazards associated with weight-loss pills. Some people spend hundreds or even thousands of dollars on supplements that don't work.

Myth #1: Muscle turns to fat when you stop exercising.

Truth: It is possible for a small portion of muscle to be consumed by the body and stored as fat. HOWEVER, the vast majority of muscle loss one might experience results from the body breaking down the muscle to consume it as readily available fuel. Muscle tissue is easier for the body to utilize than fat stores because of its protein state. If you are not doing some form of strength training exercise to maintain the muscle mass you have, the body will eventually use the muscle for energy, resulting in Muscle Atrophy.

Myth #2: Strength Training will make me bulky.

Truth: Why is it that people tend to be arrogant enough to think 6 months of strength training turns them into Arnold Schwarzenegger? I've even heard some people believe it changes your voice. Bodybuilders, power lifters, and other athletes train with great intensity for years to achieve the size and strength they do. How can one realistically believe that a moderate strength training program conducted 3 days a week will do the same as a multi-year, high intensity program?

Bottom Line: Challenge your perception when you look in the mirror. Don't get me wrong; some people are gifted with great potential for muscle growth. Notice I said some. Remember, whichever exercise you do will be enhanced by, or detracted from, the lifestyle you have. For example, if you eat too much, eat out frequently, consume too many calories, or suffer from sleep deprivation, you will have a more difficult time achieving the weight management goals you have set.

Myth #3: I need to eat a special diet to maximize any exercise program.

Truth: First, define "special" for me. Simply eat reasonably from the four food groups. What is reasonable, you might ask? Of course "reasonable" varies among individuals. When many of us were teens, we could eat an entire pizza at one sitting. Our activity levels and growth rates, needed the calories. Whatever your fitness level is at age forty, I guarantee eating an entire pizza for lunch is not reasonable when trying to lose weight. We have all heard so many plans that are billed as the "Best" for us. Ok, I agree studies have shown that more active people need a little more protein. On the other hand, some studies suggest no dieting change is necessary, except when you are trying to grow. The more complicated you try to make your new lifestyle, the less likely you are to stick to it. Listen to the Surgeon General: eat right, eat rounded meals, and eat less if weight loss is your goal. There is a fine line between eating less and deprivation; so, be careful. As with most things in life, it can be as simple, or as difficult, as you make it.

Myth #4: If I stop exercising for a week or two, I will lose everything I have built.

Truth: When you have the flu, and you cannot eat or drink as much as in a normal healthy week, do you lose all your unwanted pounds and inches? Of course not....

You will lose some, but rarely all of it over just a few weeks. Yes, you may feel a bit weaker the first day back in the exercise routine. On the other hand, sometimes it was a badly needed rest, and you comeback feeling stronger. Many of us have experienced both at different times.

Myth #5: I need to lose the unwanted pounds before I start strength training.

Truth: Muscle burns fat. Fat does not burn fat. If you want to expend more calories, you need more muscle on your body. Baring health concerns about extreme obesity, what is more important to you, your shape or the weight? Nearly 100% of my clients have said "shape" was most important. If all the unwanted—unnecessary fat were redistributed to muscle, would you be happy? Probably. Cardiovascular exercise and strength training are combined in a program to compliment one another. After all, a few more compliments in our day are something we all could use.

Myth #6: If I can just do a few more exercises for my stomach, I can lose the pooch I have.

Truth: Last on, first off! If the pooch you have was the latest place you started to deposit fat stores, it will be the first off, as you get back into the shape you desire. However, if you have had the pooch for a long time and have been putting on fat in other areas, that pooch may be the last to go. So, how do we get the fat off the fastest?

The fastest way to effect shape change is to exercise the largest muscle groups. They have the greatest potential for burning calories. If you look at an anatomical chart, you will clearly see how small the abdominal muscle group is, compared to the muscles of the legs, back or chest. Imagine the leg muscles are 20 pounds of your body and your abdominal are 3 pounds. Which group of muscle is burning more calories? Just doing the math, the legs are burning more than 6.5 times more calories than the abdominals. The fat around your waist is just another place for depositing fat. The body will use the deposit of fat to get any physical work done. If your waist fat deposit is the latest place the body has decided to deposit fat, it will be the latest place the body removes fat, when it needs energy. If it is the first place you began noticing increased size, as you became heavier, it will be the final spot the body draws fat from. I am sorry, if that is not the news you wanted to hear. This is where we stop living in denial of how the body operates. This is basic physiology. One of the first rules in life should be, to not worry about the things you cannot change, but to focus on what you can. That sentiment is so unoriginal and yet SOOO true.

Chapter 11

Fitness Fanatic

We have all seen them—those gaunt, emaciated tireless exercisers that seem to suck the life out of the room. The more casual exerciser might feel intimidated or feel just too tired from simply watching this "exercising machine" in clothes work feverishly through grueling routines. Often times, however, these are driven Type As. They apply themselves to everything as they do exercise. It is common to see this individual with the same facial intensity wearing a suit and tie as wearing running shorts and a T-shirt. The Fitness Freak (FF) typically has had a series of overuse injuries, nagging pain, and possibly is recovering from knee surgery. They are usually well educated, have white-collar jobs, and are trying to loss themselves in the exercise—escape. Often times the FF is the type of person how needs no drugs to run like a racehorse and could take any depressant and still keep coming.

If you find yourself beginning to fall into this category, I will tell you to slowdown or you will fall down. The body might be the most amazing machine in the world, but even it needs to stop long enough to tighten-up the screws. We must all stop and take physical inventory, before realizing our true physical potentials.

When is it too much. You have been given a plan. Hopefully, you have found the motivation. What is required now is the appropriate temperance. I have seen too any people finally figure out the key to this whole exercise thing, only to fall to injury.

Conclusion

New Year's Resolutions

So, I sit waiting to see the final scene of this movie. As I watch, I wonder how the main character learned of his destiny. How did he KNOW the best path for him? How did he gather strength around a message to bring it to fruition? I am left hoping, as are millions of us, that God's plan is shown to in a way which will be easily understood. Be true to the Lord and he will be true to you, a friend once told me. My friend had just left. I sat sober and alone. Once again, I put in my movie of inspiration and thought way too much. As the closing credits ran, I heard, "I am leaving on a jet plane...don't know when I will be back again." It was the dawn of my 400th day of celibacy. With my heart feeling rejected and alone, I some how gave thanks. It was a time of learning. I learned to trust in my instincts. Perhaps my instincts were merely God's message to love as is true to you and your love. I sat contemplating my resolutions for the new millennium. Some resolutions were clear, definable and came with step-by-step approaches; all the while, other resolutions where waiting definition. Although I was still nursing a wounded heart, I now knew my heart would heal. I was physically stronger, and my mind was finding peace in the present, while awaiting the future. I could not have made it this far without the effort I had pursued and persevered through, without seeing a goal or without faith.

I had trouble defining other goals, in the beginning. For instance, my goal for moving-on and letting go of my marriage put me in a quandary. How does one go about it?

As healthy as I was physically feeling, I still had emptiness. I would have capsized a long time ago, if I had not nurtured my physical and spiritual self. For me, the experience had opened many doors of learning and doorways to people I learned from.

I told a friend, who had just finalized a divorce, how much trouble I was having letting-go of my bride. My friend told me to remember that I was not letting go of the woman I loved, or the mother of our child, rather the verbal abuse and lack of respect. When I heard this, it was like a light turned on. I could see this point. There were traits I still loved about my former wife, while other traits were insurmountable issues. Even better, I found yet another moment of inspiration and motivation. Moments like this should not be overlooked, passed-over, belittled, or otherwise forgotten. Most of the time motivation comes in very small packages. As the tulip bulb grows to a beautiful flower, from what seemed lifeless, a moment of inspiration can grow our hearts well beyond our imaginations.

...and so it is with you, change what you can. You are the only person you can change. It is time to let go of who you were, face who you are, and BE BETTER. "Be better, you say? That is easier said than done," is a typical response. Well of course it is. Nothing could be more true. For the parents in the audience, how many times have we told our children not to whine? So I say to you, stop whining! If it were easy, wouldn't everyone be better? If it were easy, wouldn't you already be better? If it were easy, there would be little satisfaction in the end result. We usually take for granted our gifts and scorn our shortcomings.

You can be the exerciser you want to be, feeling better, looking better and being better balanced. Try not to get mired in how you have acted or what you have not done. Take a lesson from old Mr. Scrooge—what matters most, is what you do today.

This book is a planning process for maximizing your physical potential. Always remember that the plan is designed to clear the path. Some might just start doing something physical. "Just do it", is a great slogan at times. But if this has been your theory in the past, and you have never been able to stick to a consistent exercise program, this should tell you something. Perhaps the next time, you should have a plan that can bridge the gaps in your exercise routine. Stop telling yourself, or your trainer, that you have never been able to stick to a consistent exercise routine. I would bet that you have been able to stick to many routines in your lifetime. Perhaps they have been less noble routines, like going "Clubbing"(going from night club to night club) with friends a few evenings a week. The routines we stick to, we have prioritized. No one is perfect. Thus, I will not frown on you for prioritizing something other than caring for your physical self. Nor will I let you whine about it. When your priorities change, for whatever reason, apply what has been presented here.

I submit this from the book, *If life is a Game, These are the rules*, "Treat your body with difference and respect, and it will respond accordingly. Listen to your body and its wisdom; it will tell you what it needs if you ask, listen, and take heed."

I am still waiting for the next round of my motivation. I have found, motivation will wax and wane, as the ocean tide. If you understand this ideal, your valleys are less deep and your oceans less broad. But, keep on the look-out for moments of inspirational commitment to your priorities. When you give-over yourself—truly commit, stopping you is hard to do. When the feeling hits you, take it to the "emotional bank". There comes a time when you must make a final decision. Yet, the finality of any decision only comes through time and commitment to the decision made. The toughest thing in life is upholding a promise that one has made to one's self. When we are the only ones who can hold us accountable, the promises we make to ourselves are the easiest to rebuke. Your promise may be to eat less, exercise more, love better or be a better parent. Always try hardest to keep promises you have made to yourself. I believe you, and those around you, will gain the most from keeping these promises. I believe today is the best time to finish what you started, or start what you want to begin. As a friend told me once, "…live with your choices." The correct choices we make in life are the easiest to live with. The toughest choices are the hardest to live with. Begin any new effort, exercise or otherwise, with the words "I will" rather than "I'll try". Sure, failure is possible. I believe that if you begin with ideal that success is the only option, your chances of success are improved. Do not live with your bad choices; rather, live through, despite and beyond them.

End

Glossary

Throughout this book we will be using terms often used in exercise related environments. Becoming familiar with these terms early can make the reading move much more quickly.

Aerobic—exercise when the muscles utilize oxygen as the primary fuel source. Imagine you actually run longer than 30 seconds. Your body will need to replenish the oxygen in the muscle to keep going. If you are "sucking-wind" and have to stop, your muscle could not get enough oxygen fast enough. Therefore, if you can keep going, your muscles are getting enough oxygen.

Anaerobic—without oxygen—through 30 seconds or less. Figure it out from the above.

Cardiovascular exercise—any activity that involves exercising the heart through aerobic exercise. This refers to the focus of the work being on the cardiovascular system (the heart, veins, arteries and lungs.)

Cool-down—the period used to allow the heart rate to fall to more resting levels. As an example, if you run a sprint and stop suddenly, you may feel light-headed. The blood of the body flows to the areas of the body that have the demand. In this case, those areas are the legs. The light-headed sensation comes from the blood pooling in the legs and not returning the head fast enough. The Bottom-line is to keep moving until your heart rate gets near or below 100 beats per minute (as a general rule). Everyone is different, so heart rates vary, as does the time it takes to cool-down.

Dumbbells—It is not the person teaching you to exercise. The small hand-held bar with knobs on the ends.

Duration—time spent in the particular activity when the muscle is working. This does not include the time spent between sets resting

Free Weights—anything you lift that is not connected to or guided by a machine. In a less traditional sense, groceries are free weights.

Hypertrophy—generally, it is muscle growth. Don't worry about the real physiology.

Intensity—how hard you are working. In cardiovascular work, we usually are referring to exercise heart rate or the rate of perceived exertion. While in strength training, we are referring the resistance and your ability to lift it for a number of repetitions. For example, a high intensity strength training program usually involves heavier weights (resistance) with few repetitions

Interval Training—periods of exercise followed by periods of rest, completed in a series. Interval training is usually applied to aerobic work such as running or in an exercise class. Usually the repetitions are higher and the rest periods are brief.

Isometric—when there is a flexing of muscle with no movement of a joint or range of motion

Isokinetic—the resistance adjusts to keep the speed of movement constant. This is usually only possible with a machine using a compensating mechanical resistance. This type of training is usually seen in rehabilitation programs.

Isotonic—your traditional strength training in which you work through a resistance through a range of motion—be that resistance a soup can, an elastic band, machine weight or free weight.

METs—This is an expression of energy cost (metabolic equivalents)

Over-training—breaking-down rather than building-up; usually as a result of improper rest intervals between exercise sessions

Partial Rep—any range of motion that is less than the maximal capability of the respective joint or joints being applied. Sometimes, trainers will refer to a full range of motion like it is the only option. There are certain scenarios where a full range of motion could be detrimental to the joint being applied. As an extreme example, for someone recovering from a hip replacement, the full range of motion could cause damage to the joint. Many of us will never notice a difference in development, if we cut it short on the range of motion.

Program Development—program development is an ongoing process of evaluation and reevaluation of exercise goals based on the progress of the individual's level of conditioning

Reps—repetitions—the number of times you do something

Resistance—for this book, it is anything your work against causing your muscles to flex

RPM—repetitions per minute—or in cycling, revolutions per minute

Set—a group of repetitions with no rest between

SPM—sets per minute

Strength Training—exercise through a resistance aerobically

Toning—any exercise one does to strengthen the targeted muscle,

Trainer—the individual that is directing the exercise session. In sports, the athletic trainer usually helps care for injuries through on the field care and rehabilitation

Warm-up—any light activity that raises the core temperature of the body to prepare it for a more rigorous activity

Now you have the basic terminology again. You probably have heard these terms. Need I say it? If you don't understand any of the terms listed above, read them again. If you still don't understand, call me or talk to another professional in exercise science.

References

Acker, J. E., Jr. "Psychological Aspects of Cardiac Rehabilitation." *Advances in Cardiology: Cardiac Rehabilitation*, 24 (1978), p. 116.

Barnard, R.J. "Long-term Effects of Exercise on Cardiac Function." *Exercise and Sport Sciences Review*, 3 (1975), pp. 113-133.

Cohen, Sheldon, et al. *Behavior, Health, and Environmental Stress*. New York: Perseus Publishing, 1986.

Cohen, Sheldon, et al., ed. *Measuring Stress: A Guide for Health and Social Scientists*. New York: Oxford University Press, 1998.

Domar, Alice. *Self-Nurture: Learning to Care for Yourself as Effectively as You Care for Everyone Else*. New York: Viking Penguin, 1999.

Domar, Alice, and Henry Dreher. *Woman: Using the Mind-Body Connection to Manage Stress and Take Control of Your life*. New York: Doubleday & Company, 1997.

Freolicher, V., et al. "Physical activity and coronary heart disease." *Cardiology*, 65 (1980), pp. 153-190.

Hackett, T.P., and N.H. Cassem. "Psycological factors related to exercise." *Exercise and the Heart*, (1978), p. 223.

Haskell, W.L. "Physical activity after myocardial infarction." *American Journal of Cardiology*, 33 (1974), pp. 776-783.

Hellerstein, H.K. "Relation of exercise to acute myocardial infarction." *Circulation*, 39-40 (1969), pp. 124-129.

Kavanaugh, T., et al. "Depression following myocardial infarction: The effects of distance running." *Annual New York Academy of Science*, 301 (1977), p. 1029.

Lamb, David R. *Physiology of Exercise Responses & Adaptations*. 2nd ed. New York:
MacMillan Publishing Company, 1984.

McPherson, B.D., et al. "Psychological effects of an exercise program for post-infarct and normal adult men." *Journal of Sports Medicine and Physical Fitness*, 7 (1978), p. 95.

Ornish, Dean. *Dr. Dean Ornish's Program for Reversing Heart Disease*. New York: Random House, 1995.

Paterson, D.H., et al. "Effects of physical training on cardiovascular function following myocardial infarction." *Journal of Applied Physiology*, 47 (1975), pp. 482-489.

Peeke, Pamela. *Fight Fat After Forty: The Revolutionary Three-Pronged Approach That Will Break Stress-Fat Cycles and Make Your Health, Fit and Trim for Life*. New York: Viking Penguin, 2000.

Ratey, John J., and Catherine Johnson. *Shadow Syndromes*. 1st ed. New York: Bantam Books, 1998.

Sim, D. N., and W.A. Neill. "Investigation of the physiological basis for increased exercise threshold for angina pectoris after physical conditioning." *Journal of Clinical Investigation*, 54 (1974), pp. 769-770.

Stern, M.J., and Cleary P. "National Exercise and Heart Disease Project: Psychological Changes observed during a low level exercise program." *Archives of Internal Medicine*, 141 (1981), p. 1463.

Appendix

Here are some programs that have worked well for others in the past. Generally speaking, for most beginners, there are some key ingredients for every basic program. At times, you may find that your program may look very similar to many new exerciser programs. As you can imagine, this is the case because, most beginners start at similar fitness levels—Not Fit.

A key ingredient to most programs is a good cardiovascular base. That is to say, one must get the heart, lungs and vascular system conditioned to carry oxygen better—faster and more efficiently. This is a basic concept to exercise physiology. The biggest difference between programs lies in what people's goals are, and what they physically are able to do.

For some beginners, like Jane, she only wanted to walk at first. We outlined the general paces she may be interested in.

Jane (Walking)

	Intensity	Weights	Sets	Repetitions	Day
Exercises					
Strength					

	Resistance	Duration	Speed	Day
Cardiovascular				
Walking: 12min/mi			5mph	
15min/mi			4mph	
17min/mi			3.5mph	
20min/mi			3mph	
24min/mi			2.5mph	

Allen was interested in a very simple approach to exercise. We gave him a Hershel walker approach to his program. When Hershel Walker was a young athlete, he used to lose to his athletic sister whenever they would race. He spoke to a very wise coach that told him, you get faster by running faster—If you want to get better at running then run. Similarly, if you want to get stronger, pick-yourself-up. Do the basic exercises, and do them often. This is what Allen began doing.

Allen (11)

	Intensity	Weights	Sets	Repetitions	Day
Exercises					
Strength					
Squat Jump		body wt.	3	15	MWF
Pull-up		body wt.	3	15	MWF
Push-up		body wt.	3	15	MWF
Dips		body wt.	3	15	MWF

	Resistance	Duration	Speed	Day
Cardiovascular				
Aqua Jogging	water	50min	Interval	MWF
Walking	none	1hr	15min/mi	T Sa
*				
*				

Some more advanced programs are for those who have been consistent with their exercise. **Jody** was on a plateau in her development. We challenged her by adding sets and days to her program. She only would exercise each major body-part one-day a week, doing it very intensely.

Jody (10)

Exercises	**Intensity**	Weights	Sets	Repetitions	Day
Strength					
Squat			3	10	M
Leg Press			3	10	M
Leg Extension			2	10	M
Leg Curl			2	10	M
Abdominals			3	10	M
Row			3	8	W
Pull-down			3	10	W
Pull-ups			2	10	W
Straight-bar curls			3	8	W
Machine Curl			3	8	W
Dumbbell Curl			2	6	W
Bench Press			4	5	F
Incline Press			2	8	F
Incline Fly			2	8	F
Dips			3	12	F
Tricep Ext.			3	10	F
Abdominals			3	12	F

	Resistance	Duration	Speed	Day
Cardiovascular				
Elliptical exercise	4	30min		TTh
Cycling/Indoor	5	15min	75rpm	MWF
Interval Running	body wt.	20min	90%/2min	2/month

Debbie was looking for the next level of progress. This routine allowed her to still exercise as often as she liked without the fatigue associated with doing too much. If she had attempted to strength train each of her major muscle groups more than 3 days per week, she would have easily experienced over-training. Over-training, as we have said, can lead to emotional fatigue as well, not to mention injury.

Debbie (9)

Exercises

	Intensity	Weights	Sets	Repetitions	Day
Strength					
Squat			3	10	M
Leg Press			3	10	M
Leg Extension			2	10	M
Leg Curl			2	10	M
Abdominals			3	10	M
Row			3	8	W
Pull-down			3	10	W
Pull-ups			2	10	W
Straight-bar curls			3	8	W
Machine Curl			3	8	W
Dumbbell Curl			2	6	W
Bench Press			4	5	F
Incline Press			2	8	F
Incline Fly			2	8	F
Dips			3	12	F
Tricep Ext.			3	10	F
Abdominals			3	12	F

	Resistance	Duration	Speed	Day
Cardiovascular				
Elliptical exercise	4	30min		TTh
Cycling/Indoor	5	15min	75rpm	MWF
Interval Running	body wt.	20min	90%/2min	2/month

My son's middle name is **Jerrett**. When I met this young man, I thought of my son and the program I might give to him. Jerrett wanted results as much as anyone. He had been a victim of over-training when he came to me to develop a new routine. His student schedule allowed him to spend more time in the fitness program. If you have not guessed, I like it when people work hard and don't complain. This young man was a worker, not afraid of a little muscle soreness. He was so intense we had to teach him to listen to his body. Before coming to the fitness center, he often tried to work through soreness. He quickly learned that his results came faster and with less soreness, when he took more time off.

Jerrett (8)

Exercises	Intensity Weights	Sets	Repetitions	Day
Strength				
Squat		3	10	MF
Leg Press		3	10	MF
Leg Extension		2	10	MF
Leg Curl		2	10	MF
Abdominals		3	10	MF
Row		3	8	T Sa
Pull-down		3	10	T Sa
Pull-ups		2	10	T Sa
Straight-bar curls		3	8	T Sa
Machine Curl		3	8	T Sa
Dumbbell Curl		2	6	T Sa
Bench Press		4	5	W Su
Incline Press		2	8	W Su
Incline Fly		2	8	W Su
Dips		3	12	W Su
Tricep Ext.		3	10	W Su
Abdominals		3	12	W Su

	Resistance	Duration	Speed	Day
Cardiovascular				
Eliptical exercise	4	10min		WTh
Cycling/Indoor	5	15min	75rpm	MTThF
Stair Climbing	4	10min	30spr	MW
Interval Running	body wt.	20min	90%/2min	2/month

Cindy only had about 30 minutes a day to exercise. She wanted to get the most work possible in a short amount of time. This program allowed her to get in and out of the center in about 45 minutes, which included changing time. She worked the major muscle groups and became a fat burning machine. I was very proud of the inches she lost and the endurance she showed.

Cindy (7)

Exercises	Intensity	Weights	Sets	Repetitions	Day
Strength					
Leg Press			3	12	MTh
Leg Extension			3	12	MTh
Leg Curl			3	12	MTh
Abdominals			3	12	MTh
Pull-down			3	10	TF
Row			3	10	TF
Chest Press			3	10	TF
Fly			3	10	TF
Shoulder Press			3	10	TF

	Resistance	Duration	Speed	Day
Cardiovascular				
Cycling/Indoor	35%	25min	75rpm	W Sa

When I set-up programs, I have to listen to what that person thinks is their priority. For **Lindsey**, she liked feeling strong for her cardiovascular exercise portion, so she did that first. She wanted to have a stronger stomach and better shoulders. She also wanted to spend as little time in the fitness center as possible. So I gave her that program. I also reminded her of the bodies ability to spot-train, but not spot-reduce.

Lindsey (6)

	Intensity	Weights	Sets	Repetitions	Day
Exercises					
Strength					
Shoulder Press			4	10	MWF
Abdominals			4	12	MWF

	Resistance	Duration	Intensity	Day
Cardiovascular				
Water Aerobics		1hr	75%maxHR	MTThF

Basic Bobby was like so many beginners. He wanted the same routine each time he came-in so he could learn it quickly, and not have to walk through the gym constantly referring to his exercise card. Many new exercisers, don't want to look new. I told him to not worry about looking like he did not know what he was doing. Most people who look like they know all, make it-up as they go. I asked him if he was there to impress the "Gym Rats", or his new bride.
He got it right and found wonderful results even if he occasionally looked at hi workout form.

Bobby (5)

Exercises	Intensity	Weights	Sets	Repetitions	Day
Strength					
Leg Press			4	10	MWF
Straight-Leg Lift			2	12	MWF
Pull-Down			3	8	MWF
Chest Press			3	8	MWF
Fly			2	10	MWF
Lateral raise			2	10	MWF
Abdominals			3	15	MWF

	Resistance	Duration	Speed	Day
Cardiovascular				
Stair Climbing	40%	30min	35spm	MTh

The staff and I challenged Jason to do something he had never done before, be honest with himself. He had never been truly honest about why he was attending our facility. He wanted to complement his running with something other than casual sexual encounters with old girlfriends.

I don't know why some people make the choices they do. He decided to go to the gym on the only two days he had available, rather than develop a strong lasting relationship with a mutual friend. We all make our choices, that sometimes, not even we understand.

He found a good maintenance program in this routine. I just wished him luck in dealing with the other issue.

Jason (4)

Exercises	Intensity	Weights	Sets	Repetitions	Day
Strength					
Leg Extension			2	8	TTh
Leg Curl			2	8	TTh
Row			2	8	TTh
Bench Press			2	8	TTh
Shoulder Press			2	8	TTh
Abdominals			3	8	TTh

	Resistance	Duration	Speed	Day
Cardiovascular				
Jogging		1hr	8min/mi	MTWTh
Cycling/Indoor	Outdoor	2hrs		Sa

Sally was ready for exercise, but lacked time. She wanted the fastest results, in the shortest amount of time. If it is, if you only have a short amount of time, exercise the largest muscle group to expend the most calories—getting the most bang for the buck.

Sally (3)

Exercises	Intensity	Weights	Sets	Repetitions	Day
Strength					
Squat			3	12	TThSa
Lung			3	12	TThSa
Pull-Down			3	12	TThSa
Chest Press			3	12	TThSa

	Resistance	Duration	Speed	Day
Cardiovascular				
Swimming		40min	*	MWSa
Jogging		30	12min/mi	TTh

Henry was ready for more after his first month in the gym. He was consistent and showed progress.

Henry (2)

	Intensity	Weights	Sets	Repetitions	Day
Exercises					
Strength					
Leg Press			2	12	MWF
Leg Extension			2	12	MWF
Leg Curl			2	12	MWF
Pull-Down			2	12	MWF
Row			2	12	MWF
Chest Press			2	12	MWF
Fly			2	12	MWF
Shoulder Press			2	12	MWF
Abdominals			2	12	MWF

	Resistance	Duration	Speed	Day
Cardiovascular				
Walking	body weight	30min	15min/mi	MTTSa
Cycling/Indoor		20min	80rpm	W

As a beginner, Phil was looking to just get started in his new life. We gave him the typical beginner routine that he could handle.

Phil (1)

Exercises	Intensity	Weights	Sets	Repetitions	Day
Strength					
Leg Press			1	10	MWF
Leg Extension			1	10	MWF
Leg Curl			1	10	MWF
Pull-Down			1	10	MWF
Row			1	10	MWF
Chest Press			1	10	MWF
Fly			1	10	MWF
Shoulder Press			1	10	MWF
Abdominals			1	10	MWF

	Resistance	Duration	Speed	Day
Cardiovascular				
Walking	body weight	30-40min	20min/mi	M Sa
Cycling/Indoor	10-20%	20-25min	70rpm	W
Stair Climbing	10-20%	15-20min	30spm	Th

About the Author

Dave baldwin is a 16 year veteran of the health and wellness industry. He has trained thousands of people to exercise and been mentor to many personal trainers. His educational background in exercise science has lead him to a professional life that allows him to know, firsthand, what motivates individuals to exercise. Dave is currently the Executive Director of the Northwest Family YMCA in Houston, Texas.

0-595-21603-X